Smashing the Core Surgical Training Interview

Smashing the Core Surgical Training Interview is a crucial roadmap through the highly competitive world of surgery, written by previous Core Surgical Training National Recruitment panel members. It provides a realistic understanding of what is expected on the interview day and how best to prepare for it.

This book provides advice on how to maximise your time as a medical student and foundation year doctor in preparing for the Core Surgical Training (CST) interview process. It covers all aspects of the interview, including how to prepare the portfolio, virtual interview etiquette, and post-interview considerations.

This book contains the following:

- More than 30 clinical scenarios and more than 15 management scenarios with model answers
- Model frameworks for structuring answers
- Information covering real-life struggles, including how to maximise opportunities as a medical student, how to publish, and how to decide whether to take an F3 year
- Insights into the diverse world of modern surgery, including women in surgery, LGBTQ issues, dyslexia and neurodiversity, and challenges faced by ethnic minorities
- A framework for international medical graduates planning surgical careers

This is the perfect preparation guide for any medical student or junior doctor with a serious desire to launch a career in surgery in the United Kingdom by smashing the CST interviews.

Smashing the Core Surgical Training Interview

A Holistic Guide to Becoming A Surgeon

Edited by

Anokha Oomman Joseph and
Janso Padickakudi Joseph

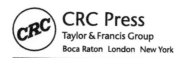

CRC Press
Taylor & Francis Group
Boca Raton London New York

CRC Press is an imprint of the
Taylor & Francis Group, an **informa** business

First edition published 2024
by CRC Press
6000 Broken Sound Parkway NW, Suite 300, Boca Raton, FL 33487–2742

and by CRC Press
4 Park Square, Milton Park, Abingdon, Oxon, OX14 4RN

CRC Press is an imprint of Taylor & Francis Group, LLC

© 2024 Taylor & Francis Group, LLC

Library of Congress Cataloging-in-Publication Data
Names: Joseph, Anokha, editor. | Joseph, Janso, editor.
Title: Smashing the Core Surgical Training interview : a holistic guide to becoming a surgeon / edited by Anokha Joseph and Janso Joseph.
Description: First edition. | Boca Raton : CRC Press, 2023. | Includes bibliographical references and index.
Identifiers: LCCN 2023009109 | ISBN 9781032388434 (paperback) | ISBN 9781032395913 (hardcover) | ISBN 9781003350422 (ebook)
Subjects: MESH: General Surgery—education | Education, Medical, Graduate | Interviews as Topic | Job Application | United Kingdom
Classification: LCC RD37 | NLM WO 18 | DDC 617.0071—dc23/eng/20230612
LC record available at https://lccn.loc.gov/2023009109

ISBN: 978-1-032-39591-3 (hbk)
ISBN: 978-1-032-38843-4 (pbk)
ISBN: 978-1-003-35042-2 (ebk)

DOI: 10.1201/9781003350422

To Dr Susmita Oomman, Thomas Oomman,
Omana Padickakudi and Ouseph Padickakudi, our parents,
for your unwavering love and support. Thank you.

And to Kimaya and Sitara, our daughters. You
give our lives meaning and purpose.

Contents

Contents

Foreword

I am pleased to have been asked to write a foreword for this useful book.

Surgery is a rewarding and worthwhile career that allows us to help and heal our patients while, for many of us, satisfying a desire to spend time, using practical skills or creating tangible innovations. This book has been written to help those taking the step up from medical student or foundation doctor to the first rungs on a surgical career ladder.

For most this is an exciting prospect, and I actively encourage it. However, having been a previous Training Programme Director for Core Surgery I am well aware of the bureaucratic and emotional hurdles that some young doctors face when transitioning from foundation trainee to core surgery trainee. There can be a minefield of information to absorb and digest. We all come from different backgrounds, and with varying levels of career foundation and support. For equitable access to training, I recognize that some will need more guidance than others.

I am delighted to see that, in addition to some very useful hints and tips on starting a career in surgery, this book touches on topics for which there is often little signposting. In particular, there is guidance for those individuals who may see themselves as being perceived as different from the mainstream. All credit to the authors for bringing these issues together in one source. We need to embrace diversity in surgery. It must be understood that people who come from different backgrounds and with different characteristics may present themselves in a different way to that which we may be accustomed to seeing, but this does not mean that they will not perform well if given the opportunity. It is diversity that brings a breadth of qualities to surgical practice and helps to build a stronger, more compassionate, innovative, and progressive profession. Without change, we cannot evolve.

I encourage all readers of this book to strive to be their best doctor, their best surgeon, and above all, their best self.

Professor Fiona Myint

Consultant Vascular Surgeon
Vice President of the Royal College of Surgeons of England

Foreword

Dear Readers,

It is my absolute pleasure to write a foreword for this book entitled, 'Smashing the Core Surgical Training Interview: A Holistic Guide to Becoming A Surgeon,' edited by Miss Anokha Oomman Joseph and Mr Janso Padickakudi Joseph. The editors have put together a wonderful group of surgical educators to write this practical and easy to read book that is filled with useful pearls for prospective surgical training applicants. Although the book is clearly focused on training programs in the United Kingdom, I think that many of the chapters contain general principles that can be applied by students around the world.

I also want to congratulate the authors and editors on writing this important book as it directly addresses feelings of imposter syndrome and stereotype threat. Now more than ever, the world needs well-trained surgeons who reflect their larger communities and will support their patients' needs and decision-making to have productive and healthy lives.

I hope that you enjoy reading this book and apply its knowledge to your own journey of achieving surgical excellence!

Roy Phitayakorn, MD MHPE FACS

General and Endocrine Surgery
Vice Chair of Education, Massachusetts General Hospital
Department of Surgery
Associate Professor of Surgery, Harvard Medical School

Acknowledgements

Thank you to the incredible authors who have contributed to this book. Each of your contributions has been rooted in your lived experience of working in surgery; this is exactly why the wisdom you share is so powerful. This book will help to close the information gap to allow candidates to succeed in securing a coveted Core Surgical Training (CST) number, regardless of their background.

We would like to acknowledge ACE Medicine and Surgery for its contribution to this book. ACE Medicine and Surgery's vision of empowering surgical aspirants with the knowledge and skills to smash CST interviews matches the mission of this book. We are grateful for an incredible partnership, rooted in deep friendship.

Thank you to Health Education England and the chair of the Core Surgery Training and Advisory Committee, JCST for clarifying that, since this book contains no reproductions of interview material, it is permissible to print.

Thank you to Virginia Haoyu Sun (Illustrator) for chapters 3, 6, 7, and 19.

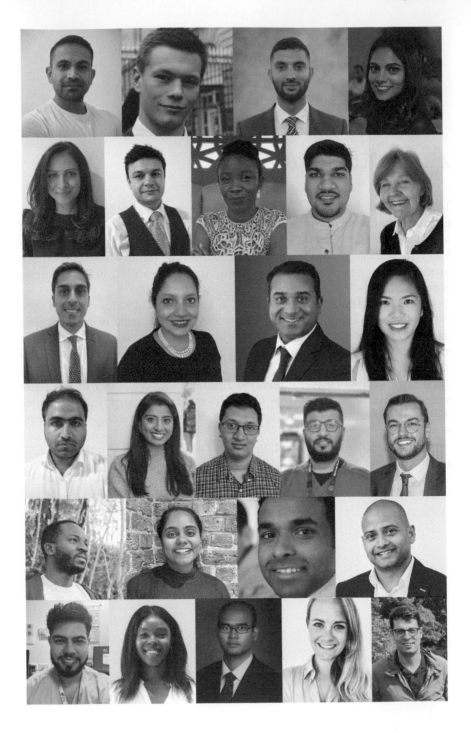

Editors

Anokha Oomman Joseph is an oncoplastic breast trainee who has completed her surgical training at the London Deanery with her final years of training at St Bartholomew's Hospital and The Royal London Hospital.

She has completed a masters in medical education from Cardiff University. She has an extensive teaching portfolio. She is a tutor for the MSc in surgical sciences at the University of Edinburgh. She has previously been an associate lecturer at Anglia Ruskin Medical School.

She is a graduate, with distinction, of the Surgical Leadership Program at Harvard Medical School. She has previously been a panel member for the National Recruitment for Core Surgical Training.

Janso Padickakudi Joseph is a minimally invasive and bariatric fellow at Beth Israel Deaconess Medical Center, Harvard Medical School (BIDMC/HMS), USA. He was a resident at Johns Hopkins Hospital, USA. He gained his CCT in general surgery from the East of England Deanery. He was awarded a Queen's Medal for Service for his work during the Ebola epidemic in West Africa.

He has completed a masters in surgical education from Imperial College London. He is currently the course lead for advanced surgical communication skills at BIDMC/HMS. He has previously been a panel member for National Recruitment for Core Surgical Training.

Contributors

Mr Goran Ameer Ahmed
Locum Consultant Oncoplastic
    Breast Surgeon
Frimley Health NHS Foundation
    Trust
Frimley Park Hospital

Dr Temitope Ajala-Agbo
Surgical Trainee
Tønsberg Hospital
Vestfold Hospitals Trust, Norway

Mr Alan Askari
Post CCT Bariatric / Upper GI Fellow
Bedfordshire Hospitals NHS Trust
Royal College of Surgeons

Miss Saarah Ebrahim
Core Surgical Trainee
Bedfordshire Hospitals NHS Trust
East of England Deanery

Mrs Tolu Ekong
General Surgery Registrar
East and North Hertfordshire
    NHS Trust
East of England Deanery

Mr Joshua Gaetos
Cardiothoracic Surgery Junior
    Fellow
Barts Health NHS Trust
St Bartholomew's Hospital

Dr Stefanos Gkaliamoutsas
Core Surgical Trainee
East Lancashire Hospitals NHS Trust

Mr Mustafa Khanbhai
General Surgery Registrar
St Bartholomew's Hospital
London Deanery

Miss Rose Kurian Thomas
Medical Student
Imperial College London

Dr Carol Leather
Dyslexia Consultant
Independent Dyslexia Consultants,
    London, UK

Mr Gopikanthan Manoharan
Post CCT Upper Limb Fellow
Robert Jones Agnes Hunt
    Orthopaedic Hospital
Royal College of Surgeons

Dr Alex Meredith-Hardy
Core Surgical Trainee
Torbay and South Devon NHS
    Foundation Trust

Mr Hari Nageswaran
Consultant Upper GI Surgery
Aneurin Bevan University Health
    Board

Dr Sushrut Oomman
Histopathology Registrar
University Hospital of Wales
Health Education and
   Improvement Wales

Miss Gargi Pandey
Core Surgical Trainee
Barts Health NHS Trust
London Deanery

Mr Haseem Raja
ENT Registrar
University Hospitals Coventry &
   Warwickshire
West Midlands Deanery

Mr Viswa Rajalingam
Colorectal Surgery
Dudley Group Foundation Trust

Mr Humayun Razzaq
Core Surgical Trainee
Aneurin Bevan University Health
   Board
Health Education and
   Improvement Wales

Mr William Rea
General Surgery Registrar
The Royal London Hospital
Barts Health NHS Trust

Ms Eniola Salau
Core Surgical Trainee
East and North Hertfordshire
   NHS Trust
East of England Deanery

Dr Muhammad Salik
Core Surgical Trainee
Aberdeen Royal Infirmary,
   NHS Grampian
East of Scotland Deanery

Miss Sharlini Sathananthan
General Surgery Registrar
East and North Hertfordshire
   NHS Trust
East of England Deanery

Miss Virginia Haoyu Sun
Medical Student
Harvard Medical School

Dr Muhammad Talha
Surgical Clinical Fellow
Nottingham University Hospitals
   NHS Trust
East Midlands

Mr Sharukh Jamal Zuberi
Core Surgical Trainee
Chelsea and Westminster NHS
   Foundation Trust

Introduction

Anokha Oomman Joseph and Janso Padickakudi Joseph

So you want to be a surgeon? You have made a great choice! A career in surgery is demanding, challenging, and incredibly rewarding. As surgeons, we are privileged to serve people when they are at their most vulnerable. The satisfaction of being able to make a direct difference in a patient's health outcome with your own hands is immeasurable.

In this book, we aim to demystify the process of becoming a surgeon in the United Kingdom. We want to empower you with the knowledge and skills to make these first steps and enter Core Surgical Training (CST). We will give you specific advice on how to prepare for the interview, both in terms of maximising your portfolio and how to approach questions systematically.

This book is particularly aimed at medical students and junior doctors who think they do not have what it takes to become a surgeon. Maybe you have internalised some common stereotypes of what being a surgeon is like and believe that you do not fit the mould. We have included specific chapters for women in surgery, international medical graduates, medical students, neurodiverse candidates, and LGBTQ candidates. There is space for you to be exactly the way you are in surgery.

We are recent general surgery graduates of the UK surgical training programme. We were interviewers for the national CST interviews and therefore have a thorough understanding of the application process. We also hold a master's in medical/surgical education. Our wonderful team of authors consists of 25 committed individuals who have lived experience of the issues and challenges they write about. We hope that our collective experience will help you in your career as you make the first steps towards becoming a surgeon.

DOI: 10.1201/9781003350422-1

chapter one

Application Process for Core Surgical Training

Stefanos Gkaliamoutsas

Introduction

Recruitment for Core Surgical Training (CST) is a national process conducted by Health Education England (HEE) London and Kent, Surrey and Sussex (LaKSS) via the Oriel online application portal. There are several key dates throughout the recruitment cycle which are important to bear in mind as late submissions are not accepted. The following table is adapted from the application timeline presented in the 2023 Core Surgical Training Supplementary Applicant Handbook.[1] This can be used as a rough guide, although there is a slight annual variation to the application timeline, and it is, therefore, important to read the relevant Core Surgical Training Supplementary Applicant Handbook[1] when it is uploaded to Oriel, usually in late October or early November every year. For example, the recent addition of the Multi-Speciality Recruitment Assessment (MSRA) exam as part of the shortlisting process and as a component of a candidate's total application score has resulted in some significant changes to the application timeline.

The Application Process[1]

Activity	Date
Job adverts appear on Oriel	By early November
Application window	From early November to early December
Invitations to MSRA	By Mid-December
MSRA dates	2-week window in January
Evidence upload dates	10-day window from late January to early February
MSRA and verified self-assessment score released	Mid-February
Interview invitations sent	Mid-February

(continued)

DOI: 10.1201/9781003350422-2

(Continued)

Activity	Date
Interview Dates	2-week window in March
Preferencing Dates	3-week window in March (overlaps with interview dates)
Initial offers made	Late March
Hold deadline	Early April
Upgrade deadline	Mid-April
Interview scores and feedback released	Early May

Applying on Oriel

Registering for an Oriel account is a very straightforward process, which you should do by October of the year prior to your expected CST start date (e.g. an applicant aiming to start a CST job in August 2024 should have made an Oriel account by October 2023).[2] Job adverts typically appear in early November for posts starting in August of the following year, with applications opening soon thereafter and remaining open for about one month. Having an Oriel account will allow you to apply for multiple specialities, should you choose to do so.

The application requires you to provide personal information, such as contact details, evidence of the right to work in the UK, and equality and diversity information. Furthermore, you must declare your employment and training history (including justification for any employment gaps of four weeks or more in the three years prior to the post's start date). You must provide details of three referees who have supervised your work over the preceding two years. Last but not least, you are required to complete a self-assessment of your portfolio for which you will be awarded points. You must ensure that you have the required evidence for any claimed achievements, as you will be required to submit this further down the application process. Once you have submitted your application, you are not able to make any further amendments, so it is a good idea to go through it a few times to correct any mistakes you may have made. Be careful not to overestimate or underestimate your points (you need to have the required evidence to back up your self-assessment scores).

MSRA

A substantial recent change to recruitment is the addition of the Multi-Speciality Recruitment Assessment (MSRA) exam, which all longlisted applicants (i.e. applicants who are eligible for a CST post per the published Person Specification[3]) are required to take and which will form 10% of the application score. If the MSRA remains part of the recruitment process for future cycles, then it is likely that invitations to the MSRA will continue to be sent in December, and the exam will be taken in a two-week period in January. The MSRA Applicant Guide should be referred to for more information on booking and sitting the exam.[4]

Uploading Evidence

The evidence upload portal opens in late January and closes in early February. Evidence needs to be collated and uploaded as one document using the Core Surgical Training Self-Assessment Portfolio Proforma[5]. The Core Surgical Training Self-Assessment Scoring Guidance for Candidates document,[6] which is updated annually, details exactly what is acceptable evidence for each category. Do not deviate from this as there is very little flexibility in this regard. Please read the Portfolio chapter for further guidance. It would be a shame to lose out on points for things that you have accomplished because of unacceptable evidence!

MSRA results and verified self-assessment scores are released in mid-February, and the top-scoring applicants on MSRA will have their self-assessment scores verified and be invited to interview. Applicants have 72 hours to submit any appeals against their verified scores, and if doing so, must explain why they feel their verified score is incorrect based solely on the evidence that has already been submitted. You will not be allowed to resubmit evidence, once again emphasising the importance of getting this right the first time!

Booking an Interview Slot

You will receive an email from Oriel with instructions on how to book your interview slot via your Oriel account. Interview slots are booked on a first-come-first-served basis. Previous applicants have often argued whether it is beneficial to book an interview early or late in the interview window. There is no clear advantage to either option; ultimately, the applicants who are better prepared are the ones who will give themselves the best chance of being offered a CST job! In terms of the time of day, anecdotally a mid-morning slot is the most advantageous as the examiners will be fresh and will have had time to calibrate their scoring with the first couple of trainees.

The CST Interview

Interviews are conducted over a two-week window in March. These are virtual and are held over Microsoft Teams with a panel usually consisting of two consultant interviewers and a lay observer, and occasionally additional administrative staff may also be present. In its current format, the interview lasts 20 minutes and is split into a ten-minute Management section and a ten-minute Clinical section. Within the ten-minute Management section, you will be asked to give a three-minute pre-prepared presentation on a topic, often relating to leadership in surgery. The topic will be emailed to you around the same time that interview invites are sent out. Following this, the interviewers will question you on this presentation for two minutes. This is then followed by a management scenario question, with five minutes allocated to answering the question. The ten-minute Clinical section consists of two five-minute clinical scenario questions.

Given that the interview makes up 60% of your final application score, it is very important to prepare thoroughly for this. The amount of time that one would need to prepare adequately for these interviews varies depending on the amount of pre-existing surgical knowledge and interview experience that you possess. Someone who has recently passed their MRCS Part A, for example, may only require a few weeks to feel adequately prepared, whereas someone who has not sat a surgical exam recently or had a recent surgical job may feel more comfortable with two to three months of preparation. Our advice would be to start preparing at least two months in advance. The first month should be spent on gathering relevant resources and revising common surgical topics.

With one month to go before the interview, the focus should shift to mock interview practice. Practising regularly under conditions that resemble those of the actual interview with a group of applicants should be prioritised. It is worth enquiring whether senior registrars or consultants at one's trust would be willing to set up mock interview sessions, as these clinicians often have experience with interviewing themselves and can be invaluable sources of information and feedback. While a lot of time will be spent revising the possible content of the interview, do not underestimate the importance of good interview techniques.

Ranking CST Jobs

You will be asked to rank jobs during the three-week preferencing window in March, during which you will also be informed of your total application score, which consists of the MSRA (10%), verified self-assessment score (30%), and interview score (60%) ranking and whether you are appointable to a CST post.

Offers are released in late March, and you will have 48 hours to make a decision. You can respond to the offer in the following ways:

1. Accept.
2. Accept with upgrades. If you chose this, you may receive an offer for a job higher on your preference list should it become available later.
3. Reject. If you chose this, you will not receive any other CST offers in this recruitment round.

4. Hold. If the offer is not accepted before the hold deadline, it is automatically rejected.
5. Hold with upgrades. If you chose this, you may receive an offer for a job higher on your preference list should it become available later. An offer that is not accepted before the hold deadline will be automatically declined.

If you choose to accept or hold with upgrades, you have the option to change your preferences by reordering them or adding/removing certain jobs, should you wish to. Be very careful when doing this, as you need to make sure you would be happier receiving one of the other jobs you have ranked above the one you have been allocated. Remember that if you are offered a different programme and are not happy with it, you cannot request your previously allocated programme back.

Accepting an Offer

If you are offered a job and choose to accept it, then you have come to the end of the CST application process. You will then be contacted by your new employer in due course with further instructions. Congratulations and good luck with the start of your surgical training!

References/Key Documents

1. CST Supplementary Applicant Handbook 2023. https://www.oriel.nhs.uk/Web/PermaLink/Vacancy/F1906CDC. *
2. Oriel Applicant User Guide. https://www.oriel.nhs.uk/Web/Resource Bank. **
3. Person Specification 2023; Core Surgical Training – CT1. https://specialty training.hee.nhs.uk/portals/1/Content/Person%20Specifications/Core%20 Surgical%20Training/CORE%20SURGICAL%20TRAINING%20-%20 CT1%202023%20.pdf. ***
4. MSRA Applicant Guide 2023–24. https://www.oriel.nhs.uk/Web/Perma Link/Vacancy/F1906CDC. *
5. Self-Assessment Portfolio Proforma. https://www.oriel.nhs.uk/Web/PermaLink/Vacancy/F1906CDC. *
6. 2023 Self-Assessment Guidance for Candidates. https://www.oriel.nhs.uk/Web/PermaLink/Vacancy/F1906CDC. *
   - *These can be found on Oriel within the "Documents" tab of the "LaKSS – Core Surgical Training – CT1, LAT1, ST1" vacancy by following the link.
   - **This can be found in the Resource Bank on Oriel by following the link
   - ***This can be found on the HEE website under Speciality training > Recruitment > Person specifications > Core Surgical Training or by following the link.

chapter two

Multi-Speciality Recruitment Assessment (MSRA)

Sushrut Oomman

In line with other medical specialities in the United Kingdom (UK), it has been announced that from 2023, the Multi-Speciality Recruitment Assessment (MSRA) will also be used for recruitment into Core Surgical Training (CST) (1).

The MSRA is a timed, computer-based exam carried out at a test centre. It is designed to assess competence at the level of a foundation doctor. It is a test already being used in other specialities, such as clinical radiology, obstetrics and gynaecology, ophthalmology, core psychiatry training, and general practice (2). Therefore, MSRA questions cover an extensive range of topics.

What Is the MSRA Used For?

The results from your MSRA will be used to create a shortlist. Only the top 1,200 applicants will be invited to interview. In addition to this, your result will contribute to 10% of your final interview score. The rest of the score will be from your portfolio (30%) and clinical and management stations (60%). Your final score will determine your rank and, in turn, affect which job you are offered.

How to Take the MSRA

The MSRA is held between January and February at Pearson Vue test centres in the UK. In situations where the candidate is affected by coronavirus, you may be eligible to take MSRA remotely using Pearson's OnVUE delivery system. This remote testing is not available for any other issue that is not related to coronavirus.

For those applying from outside the UK, local testing centres can be used. You will be sent an invite in early December to book a slot if following the submission of a completed application you are deemed to be eligible.

DOI: 10.1201/9781003350422-3

Format of the MSRA

The MSRA has two parts: (1) Professional Dilemmas (PD) and (2) Clinical Problem-Solving (CPS).

Part 1 – Professional Dilemmas

The Professional Dilemmas (PD) section tests the candidate's ability to make the most appropriate decisions at the level of a second-year foundation doctor in complex and challenging situations. Every scenario is reviewed by subject matter experts (SMEs) to ensure that the content does not contain UK-specific procedures and policies that would disadvantage candidates such as international medical graduates. There are 50 questions to answer in 95 minutes. These are situational judgement test (SJT) questions. There is no negative marking, so you should attempt every question.

There are three main domains that are covered in the Professional Dilemmas paper:

1. Professional integrity
2. Coping with pressure
3. Empathy and sensitivity

The core themes covered within these domains include professional conduct, interactions with patients, interactions with colleagues, staffing issues, prioritisation, managing workload, acting with integrity, and dealing with difficult situations in the most empathetic and sensitive manner. There is no assessment of clinical knowledge.

The possible answers listed in the question will all be realistic. The response to the scenario is compared to how close they are to the expert group's response to each question. The closer your answer is to the perfect answer, the higher your score.

The paper utilises two types of question formats. The first is the 'ranking' questions, where you will be faced with four or five possible actions, which you need to rank in order of the most appropriate to the least appropriate (1 = most appropriate, 5 = least appropriate). These are not chronological but discrete actions.

The other type of question is the 'multiple best answer' where you will be presented with eight options, and you will be asked to choose three of the most appropriate actions. These three appropriate actions when taken together should be able to fully resolve the situation.

In both these types of questions, there will be a mixture of good, acceptable, and poor responses to the situation, as judged by the SMEs. These questions do not include responses that are totally implausible.

Part 2 – Clinical Problem-Solving

In the Clinical Problem-Solving (CPS) section, each question presents a clinical scenario which requires the selection of the most appropriate diagnosis, investigation, prescribing, and management for the patient. The test covers a broad range of topics, such as medicine, paediatrics, surgery, and reproductive medicine, to name a few, and is based on the clinical practice of an FY2. Seventy-five minutes are allocated to answer 97 questions. This paper consists of MCQs (multiple choice questions) and EMQs (extended matching questions) (2).

MSRA Paper	Number of Questions	Number of Questions Contributing to Final Score	Test Time
Professional Dilemmas (PD)	50 scenarios	42 (8 pilot questions)	95 minutes
Clinical Problem-Solving (CPS)	97 questions	86 (11 pilot questions)	75 minutes

How to Prepare for the MSRA

As the MSRA score will be used for shortlisting, it is the gateway into securing an interview. You should therefore treat it as a priority. You should allocate four to six months of revision for it. This is easier said than done given your clinical commitments and other activities for CV building which you may have going on.

There are many resources available to aid in preparation for the MSRA, which include Passmedicine, Pastest, MCQ Bank, eMedica Online Revision, ARORA Medical Education, Medibuddy, and OnExamination. Once you have chosen the resource you plan to use, you should go through each topic systematically and spend time reading up on topics that you are weak in. Practice MCQs regularly in your revision period and towards the end of your preparation go through a few MSRA mock papers in a timed setting.

References

1. Overview of Core Surgery Training | Medical Education Hub [Internet]. [cited 2022 Nov 28]. Available from: https://medical.hee.nhs.uk/medical-training-recruitment/medical-specialty-training/surgery/core-surgery/overview-of-core-surgery-training/applying-for-core-training#allocation15
2. Taking the MSRA | Medical Education Hub [Internet]. [cited 2022 Nov 28]. Available from: https://medical.hee.nhs.uk/medical-training-recruitment/medical-specialty-training/multi-specialty-recruitment-assessment-msra/taking-the-msra/overview-of-the-msra

chapter three

Preparing Your Surgical Portfolio

Sharukh Jamal Zuberi, Virginia Haoyu Sun, Anokha Oomman Joseph, and Janso Padickakudi Joseph

Disclaimer: Chapter is based on requirements for the 2022 round of CST application.

In this chapter, you will learn how to collect evidence, structure, and present your portfolio to obtain maximum marks. Every year Core Surgical Training (CST) becomes more and more competitive. Therefore, every point matters. A single point can determine whether you are shortlisted, appointable, or receive an offer. It is crucial that you start collecting relevant evidence for your portfolio as early as possible; it can take longer than expected to locate and organise the required proof to present your achievements.

Before the COVID-19 pandemic, all interviews were held face-to-face. Candidates were asked to bring a physical portfolio to the interview. During the interview, examiners would review and verify each piece of evidence against the assessment criteria. In this previously interactive station, examiners had the opportunity to question candidates on any unclear evidence. This gave candidates the chance to corroborate any ambiguous evidence. Since 2021, the portfolio assessment and interview have been moved online. The portfolio review now occurs without the candidate present. This emphasises the importance of meticulous preparation and presentation of your portfolio. You need to ensure that there are no gaps in your evidence that the examiners can question. Examiners are reviewing many portfolios a day, and it is therefore crucial for your evidence to be clear, concise, and meticulously aligned with portfolio instructions.

What Is Your Portfolio Used For?

As part of the Oriel application form, you will be asked to provide a portfolio self-assessment score. Your self-assessment score is used to shortlist the top-scoring ~1,300 candidates. These shortlisted candidates will then be invited to upload evidence of their achievements to the evidence upload portal.

DOI: 10.1201/9781003350422-4

Each piece of evidence you upload will be reviewed by trained assessors. They will verify that you have claimed the correct number of points. They can change your score if they feel your evidence merits a different score from your self-assessment. This process produces your verified evidence score. After the evidence verification process is complete, the highest-scoring ~1,200 applicants are invited to attend a remote interview. A combination of your verified evidence score and interview score is used to determine your final total score and ranking (CST-Supplementary Applicant Handbook 2022).

When to Start Gathering Evidence

The earlier you start the better. If you have not yet started, the time is now! Candidates who are considering a career in surgery should familiarise themselves with the self-assessment scoring guidance as soon as possible. Looking at this document during medical school or at the start of the foundation programme can help you to focus your academic efforts during these key years. This long-sighted approach gives you the best opportunity to achieve near-full marks. If you are unsure if you want to pursue surgery, you should still collect evidence as a lot of the generic domains such as audits, and teaching experience that is required in surgery overlaps with other specialities.

Which Type of Evidence to Gather

Although each year the criteria for the portfolio change slightly, the broad principles remain the same. Your evidence needs to be exceptionally clear and precise. There is little margin for error. Examiners will not be handing you marks. We advise that you follow the self-assessment scoring guidance with precision. Any achievements declared must have been undertaken after commencing your medical or first undergraduate degree (achievements from school or before university are excluded). Once you have your portfolio together, ask a senior surgical registrar or consultant to review it. Your evidence should mirror the guidance word for word. Do not use patient-identifiable data. This includes, for example, thank-you cards or letters from patients. Hospital numbers are also an example of patient-identifiable data.

Top Ten Tips for Portfolio Preparation

1. *Aim for excellence.* Aim to pick up the top marks in each category; if you aim high, you will pick up some points on the way. Avoid zero points in any category. Every point matters.

2. *Start portfolio preparation early.*
3. *Consider the effort-to-glory ratio.* Be selective about the projects you engage with. Pick those which will get you the most marks without consuming your whole time/effort.
4. *Use your time wisely.* Consider which points are achievable in the timeframe you have left. In each domain, weigh up the time taken to reach top marks and if your time should be spent more wisely elsewhere.
5. *Work smart.* For example, in the publication domain, in the 2022 marking, the top mark (6) is awarded to the first author's original research. However, 4 marks are awarded to a first author of a case report or editorial letter, which may be more realistic for you to complete.
6. *Use your network.* Work with peers. Speak to current core trainees. Get advice from seniors. Your network will be a rich source of invaluable tips.
7. *Be honest.* If your score is significantly different compared to the assessor's score, your probity may be questioned. This can have significant ramifications.
8. *Follow the instructions word for word.* Upload your documents with the exact wording contained in the instructions. A single, succinct, complete document is best if possible.
9. *Be strategic.* You can only use an achievement to score points in a single domain. Therefore, you should use the breadth of your achievements to gain the highest points across all domains.
10. *Enjoy the process.* Putting your portfolio together will summarise all the hard work you have put into becoming a surgeon. Be proud of your achievements.

Layout

Laying out your portfolio in a structured, precise manner is key to obtaining maximum points. We recommend uploading your evidence for each domain in a single PDF file. The first page should act as a summary page, clearly informing the examiner where you are claiming points. On this summary page, you should highlight the scoring criteria, your self-assessment score, and the description of evidence in your portfolio.

Many candidates upload a single piece of evidence per domain. If you have one clear piece of evidence of which you are 100% certain that it fulfils the top criteria, then upload this. This is the most powerful for examiners. However, if there may be even an inkling of uncertainty in interpretation, you should upload more than one piece of evidence per domain within the same PDF. You should ensure that you list and present all pieces of evidence in the same order. You should highlight your name/key wording in the pieces of evidence.

Commitment to Speciality

MRCS Part A Examination

MRCS Part A is the first of two surgical exams, which you need to pass before you apply to become an ST3 in a surgical speciality. Passing the MRCS Part A is imperative for successful CST applicants. Previously candidates could gain points by simply booking the exam, but now a pass mark is required. You should aim to sit the MRCS Part A at the end of FY1 or at the start of FY2. By sitting and passing this exam you score 4 valuable points. Your knowledge will be fresh coming out of final year exams in medical school, so we recommend capitalising on this.

The two things you need to think about before signing up to take this exam are time and money. You can take it as soon as you become an FY1 doctor. Using your precious annual leave to revise is no fun, and the last thing you want is to fail on your first attempt. The exam has a low pass rate (35%) and merits adequate preparation. If you have a rotation with no/minimal out-of-hours commitment, like GP or psychiatry, we recommend using this four-month block to revise. Throughout the year there are three annual sittings for the MRCS Part A exam – January, April, and September.

Some useful resources to consider include the following:

1. eMRCS
2. TeachMeAnatomy
3. TeachMeSurgery
4. *ATLS*, 10th edition
5. Netter's *Atlas of Human Anatomy*
6. Pastest

Attendance at Surgical Courses

Surgical courses are an excellent way to increase your knowledge and skill base in surgery. Some courses are mandatory for your progression as a surgeon and may be required for ST3 applications down the line. One challenge many candidates face is the cost of many courses. Unfortunately, there is very little room to manoeuvre here. You should consider these courses as a professional investment. See what resources are available to you in your deanery; some deaneries run free or discounted courses for

Devan Johnson
126 Gower St,
London NW1 2NJ
Candidate Number 7803423

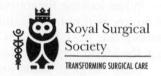

Royal Surgical
Society

TRANSFORMING SURGICAL CARE

Dear Ms. Johnson

DUPLICATE RESULT NOTIFICATION

This is to certify that the candidate attended the Intercollegiate MRCS Part A in January 2021 with the Royal College of Surgeons of England and achieved the following result(s):

MRCS Part A Result   Pass

Yours sincerely

Dr. Sam Langer
Head of Dental and Surgical Examinations, Royal College of Surgeons of England

The Royal Surgical Society
58-62 Bedford Square,
London WC1B 3JA
www.rsseng.ac.uk

Reference: 3502JC

If you need to verify this certificate, please visit www.rsseng.ac.uk/verify

Figure 3.1 MRCS Part A – pass.

their trainees. Make sure you are aware of your study budget entitlements and apply for funds appropriately.

Any surgical-themed course organised or accredited by one of the Royal Colleges of Surgeons, an international/national surgical organisation, or a deanery will be accepted. Alternatively, any surgically themed course with evidence of CPD accreditation will also be accepted. Non-accredited or undergraduate medical school society-organised courses will not be accepted. Courses that teach foundation-programme-level skills (e.g. catherisation) will not count for points.

When looking for courses, consider the offerings of all Royal Colleges of Surgeons (England, Edinburgh, Glasgow, and Ireland), trainee organisations (e.g. ASiT, BOTA, AOT), or trainee wings of national organisations (e.g. the Mammary Fold, Roux Group, Duke's Club).

Basic Surgical Skills and Advanced Trauma Life Support are particularly useful courses, conferring real-life knowledge and skills for the interview. Beware that these courses are extremely popular and can book out more than six months in advance.

Examples of Surgical Courses	Where to Book	Price (Approx.)	Length
Basic Surgical Skills (Intercollegiate BSS)	Royal College of Surgeons England	£670.50	2 days
Advanced Trauma Life Support (ATLS)	Royal College of Surgeons England	£749.00	2 days
Care of the Critically Ill Surgical Patient (CCrISP)	Royal College of Surgeons England	£799.00	2 days
Systematic Training in Acute Illness Recognition and Treatment (START)	Royal College of Surgeons England	£139.50	1 day
Future Surgeons: Key Skill	Royal College of Surgeons Edinburgh	£110	1 day
Surgical Skills for Students and Health Professionals	Royal College of Surgeons England	£99	1 day
ASIT Preparing for a Career in Surgery Course	www.asit.org	Free for members	Online
Foundation Skills in Surgery Course	www.asit.org	Free for members	1 day
So you Want to Be a Vascular Surgeon	Rouleaux Club	Free	Flexible, online
Surgical Skills	BMJ	Free	Flexible, online

Operative Experience

All candidates should create an account on Elogbook.org, the pan-surgical electronic logbook for the UK and Ireland. You should log the cases that you are involved with contemporaneously as you progress in the year.

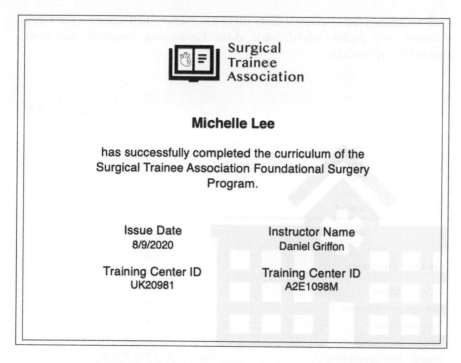

Surgical Trainee Association

Michelle Lee

has successfully completed the curriculum of the Surgical Trainee Association Foundational Surgery Program.

Issue Date	Instructor Name
8/9/2020	Daniel Griffon
Training Center ID	Training Center ID
UK20981	A2E1098M

Figure 3.2 Attendance at a surgical course.

This will ensure that you do not miss cases off your logbook. The top candidates will start doing this from medical school onwards. Your aim during the foundation programme should be to be involved in 40 cases or more for the top marks. Your involvement needs to be 'assisting' or 'supervised trainer scrubbed'; 'observed' will not count for points. If you only have one three-month surgical block in your foundation programme, you will need to participate in more than 13 cases a month. This may be difficult to achieve with your prescribed rotas. You may need to find opportunities to increase your surgical case volume. You should identify elective lists without coverage and offer to staff these. You should seek opportunities on the emergency list. We recommend involving your rota coordinator before the start of your rotation and discussing your aim for operative experience. You should position yourself in your group of foundation programme doctors as the 'go-to' person if help is needed in theatre. Many other foundation doctors will have no interest in performing this role.

The evidence for this section of the portfolio should be a consolidation report from Elogbook.org. The summary sheet needs to be signed and validated by a consultant, including their full name and GMC number. No patient-identifiable data (including hospital numbers) should be uploaded.

SURGICAL
LOGBOOK

Specialist: Min Li Chen
Date of Report : 30-Nov-2020 to 30-Nov-2021
Filter : No Filter

Consolidation Report

	A	S-TSS-TU	P	T	O	PPT
General Surgery						
Hernia - inguinal	9	9	0	0	0	0	0
Obesity - gastric by-pass	7	7	0	0	0	0	0
Appendicectomy	3	3	0	0	0	0	0
Biliary - cholecystectomy	3	0	2	0	0	0	0
Obesity - sleeve gastrectomy	2	2	0	0	0	0	0
Abscess - drainage (non-breast/anal/abdominal)	2	0	2	0	0	0	0
Biliary - cholecystectomy + operative cholangiogram	2	2	0	0	0	0	0
Biopsy / excision - skin - simple	2	2	0	0	0	0	0
Hernia - epigastric	2	2	0	0	0	0	0
Hernia - umbilical/paraumbilical	2	2	0	0	0	0	0
Obesity - lapband	2	2	0	0	0	0	0
Pilonidal sinus - excision and suture	2	2	0	0	0	0	0
Rectum - anterior resection	1	1	0	0	0	0	0
Duodenum - perforated DU closure	1	1	0	0	0	0	0
Hernia - femoral	1	1	0	0	0	0	0
Hernia - incisional	1	1	0	0	0	0	0
Hernia - laparoscopic - extraperitoneal	1	1	0	0	0	0	0
Hernia - laparoscopic - intraperitoneal	1	0	0	0	0	0	1	0
Urology - cystoscopy	1	1	0	0	0	0	0
Obesity - removal/reposition gastric band	1	1	0	0	0	0	0
Laparotomy - division of adhesions	1	1	0	0	0	0	0

Consultant: Dr. Leonard Dixon, GMC #4892409

Signature: _____   Date: 30/11/2021

Page : 3 of 4

Figure 3.3 Operative Experience Logbook – part 1.

SURGICAL LOGBOOK

Specialist: Min Li Chen

Date of Report : 30-Nov-2021

Filter : No Filter

Date	Age	Operation	Supervision	Urgency	Complications	Notes (Outcome)
09-May-2021	51	Pilonidal sinus - excision and suture	A	Elective		
09-May-2021	58	Rectum - anterior resection	A	Elective		
20-Oct-2020	33	Laser resection larynx - transoral	O	Elective		
20-Oct-2020	47	Thyroidectomy total	A	Elective		
15-Mar-2020	72	Duodenum - perforated DU closure	A	Urgent		
15-Mar-2020	66	Laparotomy - division of adhesions	A	Urgent		
23-Jan-2020	24	Abscess - drainage (non-breast/anal/abdominal)	S-TS	Urgent		
11-Jan-2020	30	Biliary - cholecystectomy	A	Elective		
08-Jan-2020	63	Hernia - incisional	A	Urgent		
02-Jan-2020	39	Appendicectomy	A	Scheduled		
28-Dec-2019	64	Appendicectomy	A	Elective		
28-Dec-2019	38	Urology - cystoscopy	O	Urgent		
19-Dec-2019	57	Hernia - femoral	A	Urgent		
15-Dec-2019	82	Appendicectomy	A	Scheduled		
15-Dec-2019	42	Obesity - gastric by-pass	A	Elective		
11-Dec-2019	76	Hernia - inguinal	A	Elective		
11-Dec-2019	58	Hernia - inguinal	A	Elective		
09-Dec-2019	37	Biliary - cholecystectomy	A	Elective		
05-Dec-2019	50	Hernia - inguinal	A	Elective		
04-Dec-2019	44	Hernia - umbilical/paraumbilical	A	Elective		
02-Dec-2019	81	Abscess - drainage (non-breast/anal/abdominal)	S-TS	Immediate		

Consultant (Block Letters) ...... LEONARD DIXON ...... **Date:** 30/11/2021 ......

Signature: ...... [signature] ......

Figure 3.4 Operative Experience Logbook – part 2.

Attendance at Surgical Conferences

Surgical conferences are a chance for you to increase your knowledge, connect with the surgical community, and showcase your work. You should attend three conferences to score the maximum marks. Many conferences are available for free or with discounted rates for medical students and/or junior doctors. You can attend these virtually or in person, with the virtual option often offering a significant discount. Single webinars will not count towards points. You should request a conference attendance certificate straight after the event and store this safely.

Examples of a few organisations that have conferences include the following. It is ideal to submit a piece of work to these conferences and combine this with attendance.

- ASiT
- Royal College of Surgeons

- Association of Surgeons of Great Britain and Ireland (ASGBI)
- Association of Upper Gastrointestinal Surgery of Great Britain and Ireland (AUGIS)
- Royal Society of Medicine
- ENTUK
- ACE Medicine
- British Orthopaedic Association
- British Association of Plastic Reconstructive and Aesthetic Surgeons (BAPRAS)
- British Association of Urological surgeons (BAUS)
- Society of British Neurological Surgeons
- Vascular Society

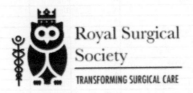

Royal Surgical Society

TRANSFORMING SURGICAL CARE

This certificate confirms that:

Tyler Sakamoto

Attended the Royal Surgical Society Surgical Conference held on 2nd-5th March 2021.

Joyce Fisher, MD
President, RSS

RSS – *transforming surgical care*
183 Hornton St, London W8 7NT, UK
555-708-2091 www.rsseng.ac.uk

Figure 3.5 Surgical conference attendance.

Surgical Experience

If you have a surgical placement during your foundation programme, you will score full marks in this section. As you are interested in surgery, it is imperative that you rotate through a surgical block to consolidate your interest. At the end of your rotation, you should obtain a signed letter from your educational supervisor on official letterhead, including the name of the placement, hospital, and the dates undertaken. Alternatively, you can obtain full marks in this section if you have completed a four-week surgical elective during medical school. If you do not have a surgical rotation you must arrange for a five-day taster week in surgery. These days can be non-consecutive. Double-check the guidelines for the exact wording and requirements required for these letters. You may need to pre-draft them for your supervisors to sign to make sure they are worded appropriately.

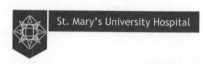

November 24, 2021

To Whom It May Concern,

RE: Confirmation of Surgical Placement during Foundation Training

I can confirm as Peyton Frank's Educational Supervisor during their Foundation Year Two training that they completed two surgical placements during their time at St. Mary's University Hospital. The exact dates are as follows:

Foundation Year One
2019-2020
General Surgery: 04-Dec-2019 to 31-Mar-2020

Foundation Year Two
2020-2021
General Surgery: 07-Apr-2021 to 03-Aug-2021

Total time spent in surgery during foundation training: 34 weeks

Many thanks,

Wendy Patel

Wendy Patel
Educational Supervisor
GMC #8087321

Figure 3.6 Surgical placement letter.

Oakland University School of Medicine

16th December 2020

To Whom It May Concern,

I can confirm that Christopher Smith completed a 3-week elective commencing from the 27th of May to 14th of June 2019 in the Plastic Surgery department at Oakland University Hospital.

Mr. Smith had the opportunity to work closely with our surgeons, following the patients journey before, during and after their cosmetic procedures. This meant that his time was split between observing theatre sessions and being part of client consultations.

In addition, he was able to scrub in and assist in a few procedures, most notably two surgeries:
- Liposuction of the abdomen
- Upper and Lower Blepharoplasty

During Mr. Smith's time he took initiative, adding relevant questions while being able to slot into the team.

It was a pleasure to work with Mr. Smith as he was polite and eager to learn.

We would not hesitate to have him again in the forcible future.

Kind Regards,

Laleh Almadi, MD
Educational Supervisor
GMC #4059283

Figure 3.7 Surgical elective letter.

Postgraduate Degrees and Qualifications

In previous years, additional postgraduate degrees were considered for points. This has been removed for the 2023 intake.

This was a section that many candidates struggled in. Compared to all the other sections, this part of the portfolio required the most investment of time and money. If you intercalate during medical school this can be used for points. You should pursue additional qualifications only if you are truly interested in the subject. During the foundation programme, there are part-time master's degrees (e.g. University of Edinburgh/Royal College of Surgeons of Edinburgh MSc in Surgical Sciences) that can

St. Mary's University

Upon recommendation of the Faculty, St. Mary's University does hereby confer upon

Steven Sanchez

the degree of

Doctor of Philosophy

with all the rights, honors, and privileges thereunto appertaining.
In witness whereof, the seal of the University and signature hereunto affixed,
This fifteenth day of June, in the year two thousand and eighteen.

Chairman, Board of Directors   *President*

Figure 3.8 PhD certificate.

be commenced. This course will also help you to prepare for the MRCS examination.

Prizes/Awards

This domain rewards candidates who have demonstrated excellence in their training. During medical school, you may be able to pick up one of the yearly prizes for various subjects.

In the context of Core Surgical Training, the prizes that are being considered relate to outstanding work that has been submitted to a medical meeting. Every audit, quality improvement project, and piece of research can be turned into an abstract and submitted to a conference. National meetings score the highest points, with regional meetings scoring fewer points. You should aim to submit your work to national meetings.

Keeping up with select organisations through mailing lists or subscribing to social media updates will alert you to opportunities, such as conferences, essay prizes, and other awards.

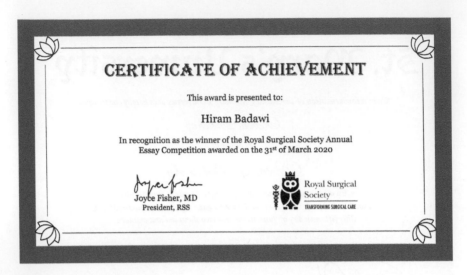

Figure 3.9 Prize certificate.

Quality Improvement/Clinical Audit

Leading a surgically themed audit or QI project that demonstrates change is a high-yield activity that can propel your marks significantly. Achieving full marks in this section can be reached by working smart. During foundation training, you must complete an audit each year. Many audit projects can come your way. It is up to you to select wisely.

Key principles to bear in mind when selecting an audit:

- Who are the registrars and consultants involved in the project? Are they known to have completed audits previously and have they published work consistently before?
- Is this a closed-loop audit – i.e. will there be a first cycle where a problem is identified and an intervention is made followed by a cycle second?
- What is the time frame? Ideally, you want to pick a project that you can finish quickly. Examples of such topics are VTE prophylaxis, antibiotic prescription, operation note standard, WHO surgical safety checklist, ward round documentation, or quality of handover.
- You do not want to be spending too long on this. You must aim to complete the audit loop cycle in less than six months.

Be careful when wording your evidence. Make sure it matches the specification word for word so there is no confusion for the examiners. In previous years, this has meant including the words 'lead', 'surgically themed closed-loop audit', and 'demonstrated positive change'.

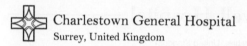

Charlestown General Hospital
Surrey, United Kingdom

December 1st, 2021

To whom it may concern,

RE: Confirmation of Involvement in a Closed Loop Surgical Themed Clinical Audit

I can confirm as one of Ms. Stephanie Parker's supervisors during her Foundation Training at Charlestown General Hospital that she was involved as a lead in all aspects of a surgical themed clinical audit that has demonstrated positive change.

Ms. Parker lead an audit titled:
'Retrospective study looking at the Standard of Safety Reports against the Royal Surgical Society's (RSS) guidelines.'

-    <u>First cycle</u>
Retrospectively analysed 70 safety reports between October 2016 – February 2020.

She presented her findings at our Local Clinical Governance meeting on the 25th of May 2020.

Intervention was to highlight awareness and create a new electronic safety report system for the general surgical team.

-    <u>Second cycle</u>
Retrospectively analysed 2 safety reports between June 2020 – December 2020.

She presented her findings at a local foundation training meeting. The results demonstrated a positive impact on the standard of safety reports against the Royal Surgical Society guidelines.

Yours faithfully,

[signature]

Michael Miller
Medical Director
GMC #2026809

Figure 3.10 Audit confirmation letter.

Teaching Experience

This section is designed to show off your teaching experience and has a big weighting. This section gives you the second most points in your portfolio. It can be a challenge to show it off accurately, and therefore, you should ensure you obtain feedback forms from students whilst also getting a letter signed by the consultant confirming involvement in designing and organising a teaching programme.

———————— Cromwell Hospital ————————

Cambridgeshire, United Kingdom
Est. 1904

December 15th, 2021

To whom it may concern,

RE: Confirmation of Involvement in the Design and Organization of a Teaching Programme

I can confirm as one of Levi Rivera's supervisors during his Foundation Training at Cromwell Hospital that he was involved as a lead in all aspects of a surgical teaching programme.

Mr. Rivera was a lead instructor in the following courses:

Tuesday Local Teaching: Designed, organised, and delivered a face-to-face teaching timetable with local educators to enhance organised teaching for Cromwell Hospital medical students at a local level. This teaching commenced on the 20th of July 2021 with more than 10 sessions. Feedback has been reviewed and deemed acceptable.

Thursday Regional Teaching: Worked with local educators (Clinical Teaching Fellows from other specialties) to design, organize, and deliver a Regional Teaching Programme Timetabled for Cromwell Hospital medical students and Montgomery University Physician Associate students. Teaching is conducted virtually to have a wider reach across the region. This teaching commenced on the 22nd of July 2021 with more than 10 sessions. Feedback has been collected and analysed from these sessions and deemed acceptable.

Students described Mr. Rivera as knowledgeable and engaging and applauded his ability to explain complex topics concisely. It was a pleasure to have Mr. Rivera as a fellow instructor of Cromwell Medical School.

Sincerely,

Yu Kyaw
Director of Education
GMC #8293841

Figure 3.11 Teaching confirmation letter.

We advise being smart in this section. Many candidates who have not organised teaching at the university level end up spending a lot of time during foundation training organising an elaborate teaching programme which may not finish in time for the application deadline.

Training in Teaching

This section is where you will show off any training in teaching you have had. However, it can be quite a challenging section to complete.

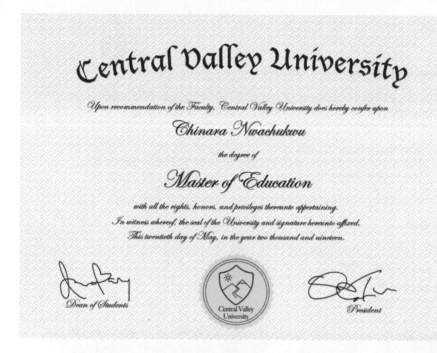

Figure 3.12 MEd degree certificate.

Many candidates will score 1 point in this section by attending the Oxford Medical – Teach the Teacher Course for Doctors, which is a two-day interactive course available both virtually and in person for £399.

Some students may opt to do a teaching-specific postgraduate qualification, such as a PG Cert or PG Diploma. However, these options are time-consuming and expensive. Moreover, if you are completing this during your FY3 year, the odds are that you will not complete it before the application deadline. Candidates need to weigh up if their time can be spent more wisely for two additional points.

Presentations

Here you should include evidence of any poster or oral presentations at international, national, and local conferences. When submitting abstracts to conferences, you should always aim for national conferences. Poster presentations are more achievable compared to oral presentations.

Typically, abstracts are derived from original research and audits. Each hospital tends to have research fellows or surgical trainees with research experience. Our advice is to contact these individuals early and express your interest. At the same time, inform them why you want to get involved in research. All surgical trainees know the importance of presentations on your CV.

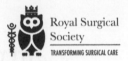

Royal Surgical
Society
TRANSFORMING SURGICAL CARE

To whom it may concern,

The following abstract was subject to full peer-review and was accepted and presented as an oral presentation for the Royal Surgical Society's Surgical Conference held on 2nd-5th March 2021. All abstracts will be published in the Journal of the Royal Surgical Society.

- **Submission number:** 1133652
- **Abstract title:** Management of Chronic Limb-Threatening Ischemia: Surgery vs. Endovascular Therapy

If you have any questions regarding the above, please contact me at info@rss.org.

Kind regards,

Rebecca Cox
RSS General Manager

Management of Chronic Limb-Threatening Ischemia: Surgery vs. Endovascular Therapy

Tracy Stewart, BS; Ada Fernandez, MD

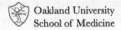

Oakland University
School of Medicine

Figure 3.13 Oral presentation letter.

A common surgical conference to aim for is ASiT as they accept a high number of abstracts.

Publications

Publications are very challenging to achieve and becoming first author of original research that is published in a PubMed ID journal can be time-consuming. We advise students to get involved in original research as first author; however, there is no guarantee that this work will be finished in time for the application deadline. Always clarify whether you will be a named author on the projects or not at the beginning.

A more achievable and realistic target is case reports and editorial letters, which are only 2 points less than a first-author publication.

A case report is a detailed report of the symptoms, signs, diagnosis, treatment, and follow-up of an individual patient. These are less time-consuming and have a greater chance of being published. The best way to get a case report is to ask your surgical seniors. Surgery is always evolving, and unexpected events can happen all the time with the on-call team or whilst in elective theatre. By being keen and asking around, you are bound to find a case that can be written up. Unfortunately, many journals now require a fee to publish case reports.

Another avenue is writing a letter to a medical journal where researchers read original papers and write a short 400-word essay as a response.

August 31, 2021

Royal Surgical
Society

TRANSFORMING SURGICAL CARE

JRSS Journal of the Royal Surgical Society
Re: MS JRSS-D-83-92013R2

Dear Avery Schuyler,

Congratulations - your revised manuscript entitled "Retrospective analysis of laparoscopic cholecystectomies during pregnancy" has been received, reviewed, and accepted. You and your co-authors have done an excellent job revising the article.

Your accepted manuscript will be sent to our production team and will be slated for publication online with listing on PubMed within about a week, and then included in an upcoming print issue of the Journal of the Royal Surgical Society (JRSS).

Thank you for publishing your work in the JRSS. Please reciprocate by contributing your expertise to the peer review process by reviewing manuscripts submitted to JRSS. We look forward to working with you again in the future.

Sincerely,

Joyce Fisher, MD
President
Journal of the Royal Surgical Society

Figure 3.14 Publication acceptance.

Leadership and Management

Many candidates have had a leadership role in some capacity whilst at university or during their foundation training. Remember that the leadership role in this section is not confined to the medical profession or medical societies. Non-medical examples may include charity, youth organisations, and sports, to name a few.

National Association
of Physician Surgeons NAPS

London, 21 November 2021

To Whom It May Concern

RE: Jaylin Hernandez Leadership role

This is a letter to confirm that Jaylin Hernandez is a member of the National Association of Physician Surgeons (NAPS).

Following an open invitation for applications and a robust selection process, Jaylin was accepted and undertook this role as of the 1st of June 2021, with their office term being one year.

Jaylin has contributed most productively to the work of the Editorial Board by:

1) Attending all meetings and appraising all issues thoughtfully.

2) Showing enthusiasm for his role by taking initiative on tasks that advance the mission of the organisation

3) Proposing new ideas and projects such as:

- Project: Comparing the efficacy of knee replacement surgeries by age group.

- Project: Do biases perpetuated in the surgical field affect medical student specialty choice?

4) Increasing the awareness of NAPS journals through his surgical teaching job.

Overall, Jaylin is a professional and diligent member of the Editorial Board with all the right attributes to succeed in surgical training.

Yours Truly,

Dr. Franklin Williams
NAPS Director of Communications

Figure 3.15 Leadership and management letter.

The key area in which individuals struggle is how they can demonstrate a positive impact. The way to showcase to the examiner that you have had a positive impact is by clearly writing a few sentences in the letter which confirm your appointment of what you have achieved during your tenure and how this led to a positive impact.

Those candidates who do not have a leadership role or want to aim for a national role can do so by applying to any national medical or surgical committee. Each committee has committee members at different levels. An appropriate and achievable role to apply for is Foundation Year Rep. We advise you to follow several national organisations on Twitter and keep an eye on when they send out applications. The more you apply, the more chance you have of getting accepted.

Conclusion

The CST self-assessment criteria are daunting to look at in the very beginning. However, as you familiarise yourself with the requirements you can build a plan for each domain. Breaking the work up into chunks can make the task more manageable; scoring points in each area is achievable. Candidates should start to work on their portfolio early, work in teams, tackle their weaker areas first, and maximise the effort-to-glory ratio.

Year after year, the overarching domains have remained broadly the same; however, the requirements within each domain can slightly differ. Each year the requirements get released a month before the application deadline, meaning there is not enough time to react to these changes. For example, in 2021, you get maximum points for a surgically themed closed-loop QI project; however, previously in 2020, the QI project could be in any speciality. The more experience and evidence you gain over the years, the more likely you are to have built a portfolio that is high-scoring despite the yearly changes.

Many candidates find it difficult to get evidence back from their consultants who are often very busy. You should take a proactive approach here. Draft a document for the consultant which matches the self-assessment criteria word for word. The consultant has the option of changing the wording. By facilitating the consultant's job, you can ensure that the evidence is fit-for-purpose and returned in a timely manner.

You should aim to score points in all domains. However, you should prioritise maximising points in sections that have the highest weight and are most achievable. This includes sections like Commitment to Speciality (20 marks), Teaching Experience (10 marks), QI Project (8 marks), Leadership (8 marks), and Poster/Oral Presentations (6 marks).

This chapter provides you with the necessary information and tools to score highly in the portfolio section. Candidates will still need to put in the time and effort to receive the required evidence. Work in a smart, methodical fashion with aim and purpose. We wish you success in your application!

Case Study: Sharukh Jamal Zuberi

I am a core surgical trainee based in London. I graduated from Imperial College School of Medicine in 2019. During medical school, I intercalated with a BSc in management from Imperial College Business School (first class honours). I completed foundation training in the Essex, Bedfordshire, and Hertfordshire Deanery from 2019 to 2021. During my second year of foundation training, I applied for Core Surgical Training with a modest portfolio score of 48/72. Unfortunately, after the interview stage, I was unsuccessful.

Instead of shying away, I used this year to become more focused on my application. I took up the role of clinical teaching fellow at the Royal Surrey County Hospital and completed a postgraduate certificate in medical education from the University of Surrey. This setback spurred me to become even more focused towards my goal of becoming a surgeon. I achieved membership in the Royal College of Surgeons of England in 2021 and reapplied for CST with a strong portfolio score of 67/72. Having achieved full marks in my interview, I was ranked second in the country during the 2022 round of CST applicants.

I am in a unique position of experiencing the very lows and highs of the application process, having applied twice for CST. In this chapter, you have read many of the tips and tricks for the portfolio section that I employed successfully.

Reference

1. https://coresurgicalprep.com/wp-content/uploads/2021/11/CST-Supplementary-Applicant-Handbook-2022-final-v.3.pdf

chapter four

How to Publish

Alan Askari

There are a few things that terrify surgical trainees more than the prospect of writing and publishing a scientific paper. At the heart of this dread is a series of misconceptions. The most inhibiting of these is that carrying out academic projects and publishing papers are inherent traits that some lucky chosen few are born with, rather than a skill that can be learnt by anyone. I hope that this chapter will dispel some of those myths and demonstrate that writing and publishing scientific manuscripts is a skill that is learnt over time, like any other in surgical practice, and is not one that is particularly difficult to learn. This chapter will focus on how to organise yourself to write scientific papers and move on to getting them published in a timely manner. At the end of the chapter, there is a template for your writing endeavours.

Myths

The preconception that writing papers is only for 'academics' in surgery is so pervasive that it has led to many trainees developing a fixed rather than a growth mindset. Many trainees only write the minimum papers require to graduate from surgical training. Over the years, I have heard many reasons that people 'cannot write a paper'. Here are my top five favourite myths:

1. *Writing papers is hard/takes a long time:* Whilst it is true that writing a scientific paper requires the dedication of time and effort (like any other new skill we learn), it is important to remember that it is not a particularly long learning curve. Maintaining momentum is the *single most* important factor in successfully completing a project. Many projects fall into the academic graveyard and are never completed for the simple reason that participants do not persevere to get over the last few hurdles despite investing weeks and months of work into it.

DOI: 10.1201/9781003350422-5

2. *I'm naturally no good at writing papers:* Strictly speaking, this is absolutely true, but guess what? No one is naturally good at writing papers! It is a skill that we learn and develop. Yes, some people may have more ability and will be quicker on the learning curve, but no one is 'naturally gifted' in writing a paper any more than they are at driving a car or playing the violin. They learn over time and so can you.

3. *I'm not a native English speaker/writer:* Whether we like it or not, English is the lingua franca of academic writing. Whilst native English speakers may find it easier to overcome their learning curve, anyone can be trained to write an academic paper. Some of the best manuscripts I have seen written have not been written by native English speakers.

4. *I can't write 'scientifically':* The idea that a good article must be lengthy and requires complicated writing to make it seem credible is quite frankly preposterous. Quite the opposite is true – the most well-written academic papers are those in which the authors can deliver the key ideas and message of their project in a style and format that can be easily understood. As one of my all-time heroes, US physicist Richard Feynman, once said, 'If you cannot explain something to a first-year student, you don't know it well enough'.

5. *Only high-impact factor journals publish well-written papers:* Impact factor, h-index, and all other metrics of measuring academic output have their own controversies. The medical literature is full of examples of how even the highest-impact journals can publish articles which have turned out to be incorrect or in some cases, even worse, outright fraudulent. Equally, some of the best, most practice-changing papers have been published in relatively lower-impact journals having been rejected by the 'big hitters'.

The Recipe

Now that we have successfully dispelled all these myths and fixed ideas, it's time to get into a growth mindset. The remainder of this short chapter will focus on a step-by-step cookbook that will have you writing in no time. Let us assume that you have completed your project, i.e. you have collected all your data, you know what outcomes you are investigating and now the time has come to write it up and submit it to a journal. Here are 10 easy steps that will help you get there quickly:

1. *Have a template:* Never, ever, ever write up an academic paper starting from a blank document. It is the most demoralising and painful experience you can have in academia and the surest way of putting

you off writing it altogether. Instead, create a template that is filled with sub-headings and bullet points that you can use for every paper. That way, when you come to write a paper, all you need to do is write around the bullet points that you have written, and before you know it, half the paper is written for you. My first session of writing a paper is only this – populating my template with bullet points, ideas, and short notes. I then leave it and come back to it at a later date to fill in those bullet points.

2. *Clarify what you want to convey:* This cannot be overstated enough; have a clear understanding, in very simple everyday language, of the message you want to convey. The simpler the language, the more direct, the better. Avoid the use of colloquialisms and unnecessary words. Remember, in science complicated does not mean better.

3. *Work in bursts:* It is very difficult, if not impossible, to write a manuscript from start to finish in one sitting. This is one of the main areas where people go wrong. They feel like they need to clear an entire weekend of their lives to dedicate to writing the manuscript. Inevitably this is not possible. Surgical training, work duties, partners, family, children, and life in general will have other plans for you. As a result, that weekend where you were going to 'just write' never comes. The project runs out of steam, months go by, and that blank document that was going to be a paper just sits there on your laptop. Be realistic. Work in bursts. Have a way of scheduling time to write just two to three paragraphs a week. Before you know it, in a month you have a paper!

4. *Maintain momentum:* This is the mother of all project killers. We have all been there. Over a coffee break after a ward round, a group of clinicians gather round, and someone will pipe up with 'It would be really interesting to look at . . .' or 'We have some data we collected, we just need someone to write it up . . .' And just like that, a project is born to applause and fireworks. Two months later, nothing has moved forward. Avoid this like the plague; at that very same meeting, write out who the project members are and who will do what and by when. Assign responsibility and realistic deadlines to each team member and hold them to account. Make them buy the coffee each time until they do not deliver; they will either stop drinking coffee with you, or you will get the project done. Either way, you will know where you stand. There are no rewards for half-finished projects. To quote everyone's favourite vertically challenged, green sage, 'Do or do not. There is no try'.

5. *Re-draft:* Accept that more than one draft is necessary. Therefore, selecting collaborators for your team is of vital importance. Different people will have different perspectives on your work. It is very easy

to develop tunnel vision when you are writing a manuscript from start to finish.

6. *Use technology wisely:* Never work with 12 different tabs open, including your favourite animals doing cute activities on YouTube. Close all non-essential programs, remove your phone to another room, and set an allocated time to write your two to three paragraphs in that one sitting. Emailing your fellow collaborators, the 14th re-draft (23 drafts is my personal record – I am still recovering from that trauma) is a terrible idea. Use cloud-based documents, such as Google Drive, Dropbox, or Box, so that everyone is working from a single document and all changes made can be seen by everyone in real time.

7. *Use a reference manager:* I remain convinced that those who do references manually must hate not only themselves but all living beings in the universe. Otherwise, why would they want to introduce so much suffering into the world? It takes hours to do references including every dash, dot, full stop, bracket, italic, boldface, and who knows what else to a particular journal's liking. Then what happens? Your consultant, attending, senior author, or professor decides actually the *International Journal of Occult Mythological Medicine* would be a better fit for your paper than the *World Journal of Occult Mythological Medicine*. Of course, they both have completely different referencing formats. There goes the weekend. Use a reference manager. There are many different ones out there. Many are free, and some require a subscription or a small fee. Examples are EndNote, Zotero, and Mendeley. It does not take long at all to learn how to use them, and it will save you hours of time and months of psychological therapy.

8. *Select your target journal:* Different journals have different interests, and they have specific readerships to cater to. Think carefully about whether your paper is something that this journal is interested in. Have they previously published similar papers? Optimism is a very nice trait, and far be it for me to discourage it, but sending your n = 15 patients who had wound complications after appendicitis to *Nature* is unlikely to yield favourable results.

9. *Respond to reviewers:* Once you do get a journal that is interested in your manuscript and asks you to make minor amendments or to respond to reviewer comments, get started on it early. Reply to each specific point raised by the reviewers in a different colour and highlight the changes in the manuscript to make it easy for the editor to identify.

10. *Be resilient:* Nineteen – yep, 19 – that is my record number of rejections for a single paper before it finally got accepted somewhere. Accept that not every journal or reviewer will like what you write.

Accept that reviewer 2 (it is always reviewer 2) will come up with some ridiculous comment that will make you question if the editor sent them your paper or someone else's. Take the good points and the advice, and make the changes that you and your fellow authors think are reasonable and send them to the next journal on the hit list.

[Title of Manuscript]

Full Names of Authors

Author Titles and Affiliations

- Relevant medical degrees of each author
- Hospitals/universities each author is affiliated with

Corresponding Author

Name and email of the corresponding author

Conflict of Interest and Funding

The authors declare no conflict of interest, and no funding has been obtained for the purposes of this study.

Author Contribution

- Report how each author contributed to the study (e.g. 'The study was conceptualised by AA and AB. Data collection was performed by AA, AC, and AD. The manuscript was written by AA and AE and edited for scientific content by AE and AF').

Abstract (200–300 words)

Introduction (1–2 lines)

- Line 1 (brief background of the main condition): Diabetes is a common chronic condition affecting millions of people worldwide.
- Line 2: The main aim of this study is to determine the efficacy of metformin in treating type 2 diabetes.

Methods (1–2 lines)

- Line 1: A systematic review and meta-analysis were conducted using PubMed, Google Scholar, and OVID.
- Line 2: The PRISMA checklist was used, and Forest plots were generated to demonstrate the difference between the two groups.

Results (3–4 lines)

- Lines 1–2: Main demographics: A total of xxx articles/patients were included in this study, of which xxx% were female; the median age was xxx years (IQR yy-zz).
- Lines 3–4: Main findings: Patients who underwent treatment xxx were 35% more likely to . . .

Conclusion (1–2 lines)

- Line 1: Treatment xxx is associated with xxx in patients with xxx.
- Line 2: The recommendations of this study are . . . Further work is required to clarify whether this is . . .

Introduction (2–3 paragraphs)

- Paragraph 1: Opening paragraph about the health condition/situation.
- Paragraph 2: Brief background on what others have reported on this specific issue.
- Paragraph 3: Explain why research in this area is important. The last sentence should lay out what the aim of the study is.

Methods (2–3 paragraphs)

- Paragraph 1: The duration of the study (e.g. 'from January to May 2015') and inclusion criteria.
- Paragraph 2: Ethical approval (if required), variables collected, and statistical analysis.

Results (3–4 paragraphs)

- Outline the key findings of the study with reference to tables and figures.

Discussion (6–8 paragraphs)

- Paragraph 1: The first line must state the main findings of the study.
- Paragraphs 2–6: The main discussion points in relation to findings of other studies.
- Paragraph 7: Main limitations of the current study.
- Paragraph 8: Summary of the paper, conclusion, and future work needed.

References

- Check journal referencing format and use referencing software, such as Mendeley, EndNote, ReadCube Papers, EasyBib.com, Zotero, and Article Galaxy Enterprise.

Tables and Figures

- Label all tables and figures.
- Limit the number of tables and figures to a maximum of five to six in total.
- Ensure tables and figures are referred to in the text and there are no contradictions.

chapter five

Mastering the Presentation

Humayun Razzaq and Janso Padickakudi Joseph

During this highly predictable part of the interview, you will need to give a short presentation about a predefined topic and answer questions for a couple of minutes. Invariably, the topic relates to a broad aspect of surgery, such as leadership, teamwork, or communication, and how this relates to being a core surgical trainee (CST). If you come prepared, you can score full marks on this aspect with ease.

Understand Definitions

Read and re-read the topic for your presentation and ensure you understand all the questions' components. When you are preparing your answer, be sure to address every part of the stem.

Imagine the topic is leadership. Make sure that you understand the definition of leadership inside out. This does not just involve the dictionary definition. Read about different ways and models to conceptualise leadership. Ask yourself the definition from a multitude of angles. For example, you should be able to answer what are the attributes of a good leader, what makes a bad leader, and what the difference is between leadership and management.

Use Your Own Experience

Now that you understand the definition, delve deep into your lived experience, and dig up the most pertinent examples that show how you demonstrate these attributes. Your examples can certainly come from medicine. However, they are often more memorable and powerful if they come from outside of medicine. Make sure that you chose an example of something reasonably recent. And make sure that it is an example that you are passionate about. This is also the time to showcase your uniqueness, and diversity in thought will be appreciated here. Imagine the situation from an interviewer's point of view. Interviewers will be hearing presentation after presentation about an individual leading a trauma team or leading a

DOI: 10.1201/9781003350422-6

quality improvement project. Of course, these can be effective and interesting. However, you will catch the interviewer's imagination if you present an example that is outside the box.

Relate Your Experience Back to CST

Once you have picked one or two examples to speak about, make sure that you flesh out what attribute you are trying to present. If the attribute is, for example, the ability to delegate, then make sure that you tie this back in with life as a CST. This will show the interviewer that you understand the realities of being a CST. You must complete this step, as otherwise you have just told an interesting story without demonstrating why this makes you an outstanding candidate to become a surgeon.

Practise, Practise, Practise

When narrating the experience, it is important that it showcases your ability to communicate effectively. There is a lot of emphasis on developing and consolidating communication skills in CST. You should aim to make no more than three points during your presentation, as it will be too unwieldy otherwise. Use top-down communication, which means setting the scene first ('In my presentation, I am going to speak about X, Y, and Z') and then delving deeper into each. That way, the interviewer has a roadmap of where your presentation is going. Make sure that you have a strong concluding sentence to avoid an awkward silence at the end. Practise in front of the mirror, to your colleagues, to your friends and family. Try your presentation on someone outside of medicine. This will give you valuable insights. For full marks, your presentation should be well-rehearsed, delivered without notes, and precisely timed.

chapter six

How to Structure Your Answers Clinical

Anokha Oomman Joseph and Janso Padickakudi Joseph

Having a logical, robust structure to your answer will allow you to present yourself as an organised, trustworthy core surgical trainee (CST). Although there is no one right way to deliver an answer, we present a scaffold on which you can build during your practice sessions. You should aim to deliver your answer in one go, without interruption by your assessor. If you answer all the points on the scoresheet through your unprompted answer, you will score maximum points.

The example scenario that we will use is as follows:

You are the core surgical trainee on the trauma team. You are asked to attend to a major trauma. The patient is a 27-year-old male driver of a car that has crashed. He is complaining of intense abdominal pain. He is haemodynamically unstable.

Step 1: Identify the problem, and mention possible outcomes.

- Usually, the stem of the question relates to one obvious disease pathology. Very occasionally, there may be two competing diagnoses. You should start by stating this clearly. Your second sentence should mention possible outcomes – usually either a scan or an intervention. By starting the case in this way, you focus the examiner's mind and let them know that you understand the big issues and decisions at hand.
- *In this scenario, I am concerned that the patient is acutely unwell and has a possible life-threatening intra-abdominal injury, such as bleeding from the liver or spleen. They may be in haemorrhagic shock. I am considering whether the patient is stable enough for a scan or whether they may need to go to theatre immediately for a damage-control laparotomy.*

DOI: 10.1201/9781003350422-7

Step 2: Alert the appropriate team.

- If you are dealing with an unwell patient, you need to make sure to alert the correct team. Sometimes it will be entirely appropriate for you to make an initial assessment independently. If the patient is severely unwell, you will want to alert the medical emergency response team, the trauma team, or your registrar very early. There is a fine balance here between working autonomously to the level of a trustworthy CST or being seen as either too cautious or overconfident. The key is to appear competent, confident, and safe.

- *In a haemodynamically unstable trauma patient with a potential for significant injuries, I need the help of the entire trauma team. I would ensure a trauma call has been put out, with all associated specialities in attendance, including general surgery, A&E, and orthopaedics. Given the severity of this patient's presentation, I would alert my registrar immediately.*

Step 2: Use an assessment framework to make an initial assessment.

- Whenever you are assessing an unwell patient, you should use a framework. In an acutely unwell patient, you should use the CCrISP model. In a trauma scenario, you should use the ATLS model. In either case, you will perform an A–E assessment of the patient initially, then look at basic investigations or documentation. The extent to how detailed your description of the A–E assessment will depend on the acuity of the patient. If you have a trauma patient who is short of breath, you want to describe the airway and breathing assessment sequentially, in great detail. Conversely, if you have a post-operative patient who is septic, A and B will not be as relevant, and you can skim over these. The key is to make a sensible, holistic assessment of the patient.

- *I would attend to this patient immediately using the ATLS approach. I would ensure that their c-spine is secured with three-point immobilisation. I would make an assessment of their airway by speaking to the patient. I would introduce myself and ask them their name. If they are able to respond, I would move on to B. I would listen to their lungs to ensure equal air entry bilaterally. I would assess their respiratory rate and oxygen saturation. I would check for significant injuries to the chest wall. I would deal with any life-threatening findings such as a tension pneumothorax at this stage. In C, I would obtain the patient's heart rate and blood pressure. If they are hypotensive and tachycardic, I would be concerned about haemorrhagic shock from intra-abdominal bleeding. I would ensure the patient has two large-bore peripheral IV lines, with blood specimens sent off at the same time, including an FBC, U&E, LFTs, coagulation screen, X-match for four units, and VBG. I would activate the major haemorrhage protocol.*

Given how unwell the patient is, I would give them two units of O-negative blood and see how they respond. Given that I believe they are having intra-abdominal bleeding, I would also examine their abdomen at this stage to see if they are peritonitic. To complete my primary survey, I would proceed to D by examining GCS, temperature, and pupils. For E, I would examine long bones and perform a log roll with rectal examination.

Step 3: Speak about the history and physical examination.

- State what aspects of the history and physical examination you find relevant. For example, in a trauma patient, you want to understand the mechanism of injury through a focused history. You will also want to localise any pain they are experiencing. Physical examination should be described, with a couple of potential findings. In the example, you have already performed most of the physical examination during the detailed A–E assessment. Here you will need to be creative about potential findings and outcomes, as the examiners will not give you any further clinical information.

- *Once my primary survey is complete and I have addressed any life-threatening complications, I would ask the patient for a focused history, including an AMPLE history (allergies, medications, medical history, last meal, events). At this stage, if the patient is not responding to resuscitation and has a peritonitic abdomen, I would be concerned about life-threatening intra-abdominal bleeding. If they are responsive to resuscitation, we may have time for further investigations.*

Step 4: Speak about investigations.

- Here you will want to discuss any investigations that can either help you make a diagnosis or a decision. You have already sent off blood tests in your A–E assessment, but you may also want to consider microbiology (e.g. blood cultures in a septic patient), diagnostic radiology (e.g. FAST scan at bedside, x-rays, ultrasound, or CT scan), interventional tests (e.g. interventional radiology, interventional endoscopy), or operative management (i.e. straight to theatre).

- *In this scenario, the patient is haemodynamically unstable. If they do not respond to resuscitation, then I would ask A&E to perform a FAST scan at the bedside. This will confirm if there is free fluid in the abdomen. This is a surgical emergency and will need to go to theatre for a damage-control laparotomy. However, if they respond well to the resuscitation and are no longer tachycardic and hypotensive, I would consider whether to get a scan. This would take the form of a triple-phase CT of the chest/abdomen/pelvis. This scan will localise the injury and potential source of bleeding.*

Step 5: Escalate/involve.

- Now that you have made a full assessment of the patient, you want to escalate their care appropriately. This includes escalating up and down within your own team. Involve your foundation doctors and any physician associates on your team, and delegate tasks to them. Escalate early to your registrar and the consultant on-call. You also want to escalate across to other medical specialities (e.g. medicine, anaesthesia, paediatrics, or interventional radiology) as appropriate to the case. You may want to involve other teams (e.g. intensive care, critical care outreach, or theatres). Finally, consider members of the wider healthcare team that require involvement, including nurses, radiographers, porters, the theatre coordinator, or the site manager.

- *When managing this patient, I would utilise my entire team. I would ask my FY1 to perform specific tasks during the assessment and resuscitation, such as running the VBG and communicating the result back to me. I would escalate early to my registrar and even directly to my consultant in this life-threatening scenario, especially if I think the patient needs an emergency laparotomy. I would want to involve other specialities early, including radiology, ICU, or anaesthesia. In addition, I will need to liaise with nursing staff or the theatre team if I thought the patient needed to go to theatre immediately. If the patient needed to go for a scan, I would alert the radiographers and porters as to the urgency of the scan. I may also want to discuss scan findings with interventional radiology. All the while, I would ensure*

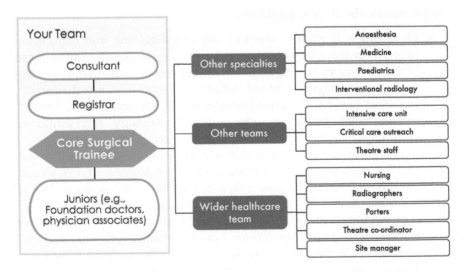

Figure 6.1 Clinical escalation pathway.

that there is a member of staff assigned to document this patient's progress contemporaneously, and I would write notes as soon as the patient's urgent needs are met.

Step 6: Keep the patient at the centre of care.

- If you can keep the patient at the centre of care while you discuss this scenario, you will demonstrate your real-life empathy. This will set you apart from most candidates. Always consider whether there are wider social issues that you be leading to this presentation – for example, is a trauma an accident, a self-harm attempt, or an assault? Are there safeguarding issues to consider? Is any long-term follow-up required?
- *Throughout all of this, I would keep the patient at the centre of care and, if possible, involve their family. I appreciate that this is a high-stakes, life-threatening situation and that this can be scary or stressful for the patient. I would ensure that their symptoms, especially pain, are adequately controlled using medications. I would also speak directly to the patient, explaining every step of the way, addressing them by name, and making eye contact with them, as it must be frightening for so many things to be happening at once while in the supine position. I would involve the patient's next of kin and keep them informed. If the patent needs to go to theatre immediately, I would consent them if I felt comfortable or, alternatively, fill out a consent form 4 if the patient was not in a state to consent.*

chapter seven

How to Structure Your Answers Management

Anokha Oomman Joseph and Janso Padickakudi Joseph

Like in the clinical scenario, you should have a logical, robust structure to your management scenario answer. For most questions, you can use the SPIES framework (seek more information, patient safety, initiative, escalate, support) to deliver your answer. If you can bring in empathy and personal experience, this will show that you are truly ready to become a CST. Again, you should aim to deliver your entire answer in one go, without the need for prompts.

The example scenario that we will use is as follows:

You are the new core surgical trainee on urology in a tertiary centre. The job is known to be busy. There are four unfilled posts on an eight-person junior surgical rota. You find that you are being asked to cover on-calls regularly. How would you approach this situation?

Step 1: Identify and name the problems.

- Once you read the scenario, take a deep breath and think. Try to distil the issues into the two or three most important management problems. You will not be able to speak about all facets of the problem, so focus on the key issues. Here you want to use big-picture buzzwords, such as 'patient safety', 'professionalism', 'training', or 'workforce planning'.
- *The key management issues are the distribution of work, patient safety, and my own training needs. I would approach this situation with an open mind as on-calls are often an excellent learning opportunity, both in terms of managing patients and exposure to theatre.*

DOI: 10.1201/9781003350422-8

Step 2: Seek more information (S).

- State how you would approach this situation and gain the maximum amount of information. Make sure that you consider your viewpoint and those of others. Be sure not to be accusatory or biased in your assessment, and approach the problem with a growth mindset – i.e. that there are important things to learn, even in a difficult situation.
- *As a first step, I would review the rota to determine if my suspicions are correct. I would see how many on-calls I have been covering and whether this has impacted other aspects of my learning. I would also assess if there have been other adjustments made because of the increased on-call frequency, such as dedicated theatre days or compensatory days off. I would review my logbook and workplace-based assessments and evaluate whether I am on track to achieving the required competencies.*
- *I would initiate a discussion with the three other junior doctors on the rota. I would ask about how they are managing their duties and weekly schedule, including time on the ward, clinics, and theatre. Perhaps there are other trainees who have previously been on this rotation. I can approach them to find out if this has been a recurring issue.*

Step 3: Consider the impact on patient safety (P).

- Everything we do in clinical medicine eventually leads back to patients. You need to centre your response to reflect that you understand that the patient is the centre of everything we do as clinicians, be that providing clinical care, teaching, or research. We recommend that you address patient safety directly.
- *My main concern is the potential impact that staffing shortages can have on patient safety. I would consider the impact of the staff shortage on the provision of services, both elective and emergency.*

Step 4: Take initiative (I).

- You should present yourself as a thoughtful, proactive team player. You should aim to make a positive contribution to whatever difficult situation is being presented to you. In a management scenario, this may take the form of an audit to further understand the situation.
- *At this point, I would consider auditing the rotas over a period of a few weeks to assimilate evidence of my concerns. I would seek out as many training opportunities in my current situation until things have been resolved.*

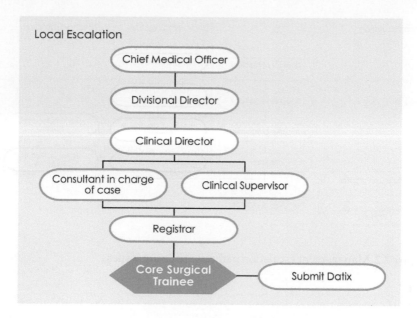

Figure 7.1 Management escalation pathway: clinical issues.

Step 5: Escalate (E).

- With the evidence in hand, you will want to escalate your concerns. Usually, this takes the shape of three routes of escalation: clinical, training, or professional. Make sure you mention every step and stop if your concern is resolved.
- The clinical escalation pathway for management scenarios is as follows: registrar → consultant in charge of case → clinical supervisor → clinical director → divisional director → chief medical officer (CMO). You will also want to submit a Datix report (Figure 7.1).
- The training escalation pathway for management scenarios is as follows: At the local level, it involves the registrar → educational supervisor → Royal College tutor → director of medical education. You may also want to involve the rota coordinator and guardian of safe working. At the deanery level, it involves the trainee representative →

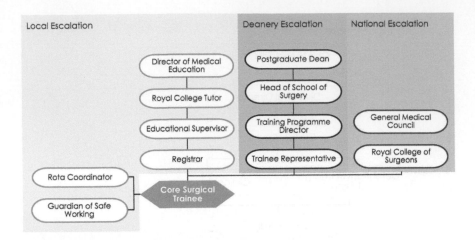

Figure 7.2 Management escalation pathway: training issues.

training programme director → head of the school of surgery → post-graduate dean. If the issues persist, you would escalate to the General Medical Council or the Royal College of Surgeons (Figure 7.2).

- The professionalism escalation pathway for management scenarios is as follows: registrar → educational supervisor → clinical director → divisional director → chief medical officer → chief executive officer. Depending on the circumstance, you may also need to involve the deanery, as detailed. In extreme circumstances, if your concerns remain unresolved, you will want to escalate to external organisations, including the BMA, the GMC, the Royal College of Surgeons, or your defence union (Figure 7.3).
- *I would escalate my concerns to my educational supervisor, my clinical supervisor, and the rota coordinator. I would try to proactively suggest solutions that have been discussed with the other junior doctors. Perhaps the fair distribution of on-calls and increased support of other training requirements are required. Perhaps foundation-year doctors or registrars are able to cover some of the duties. Maybe locum doctors might need to be recruited. The department should also consider why there are four vacant positions and how these can be filled.*

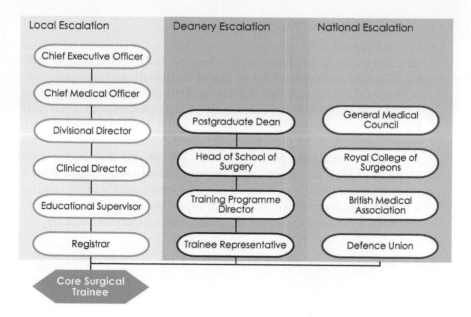

Figure 7.3 Management escalation pathway: professionalism issues.

- *If my concerns are unresolved, I would escalate them to my trainee representative or the Royal College tutor. If my training is being impacted significantly, I would involve my training program director. The clinical director for the department, director of medical education, and the guardian of safe working may also need to be involved. The British Medical Association may also be consulted, especially to ensure that the rota is compliant with the European Working Time Directive.*

Step 6: Support (S).

- You need to show empathy and concern for your colleagues, even in a scenario where you may be feeling attacked. You can demonstrate your understanding of complex situations – for example, by saying that you may not be able to provide support directly – but support may be available.
- *As all of this occurs, I would offer support to my fellow junior doctors, who may be struggling with the intensity of the workload. I would aim to manage this situation in a calm and professional manner.*

Step 7: Final considerations.

- In closing your management scenario, you want to make any final considerations. If you have not yet done an audit on the subject matter, this may your chance to say it. An audit will not be appropriate in every case. You will also want to present yourself as a thoughtful future CST and want to include reflection as part of your answer. If the scenario involves harm to a patient, you will want to apologise to the patient and direct them to the Patient Advice and Liaison Service (PALS). You will want to enter a Datix report and discuss the case at the morbidity and mortality meeting. The situation might need a root cause analysis. If you are facing a never-event, this will require a serious incident report and central reporting. You, or a member of the team, will need to inform the patient using duty of candour.

chapter eight

Virtual Interview Etiquette

Viswa Rajalingam and Janso Padickakudi Joseph

Introduction

Since the COVID-19 pandemic, there has been a seismic shift in the adoption of video-conferencing tools. What started out of necessity has now become a convenience. Video-conferencing applications, such as Zoom and Microsoft Teams, have become ubiquitous in almost every industry, with medicine and surgery being no exception. Core surgical training interviews are now web-based and seem set to be so for the foreseeable future. Understanding and mastering these applications is essential to allow you to communicate clearly and effectively and present your best self to the panellists. Before you even think of joining your first video call, you must ensure that you are appropriately set up. Most of our communication is nonverbal, so you must be seen and heard well.

The Setup

Stable Internet

Make sure that you have a stable, fast internet connection for the interview. A superfast broadband connection plugged into your device is far better than relying on a mobile hotspot. The availability of the internet or WiFi signal strength may determine where you conduct your interview, whether it is in your home, a friend/relative's home, your hospital, or your university. Prior to connecting, disable/hold off any major system updates to the operating system, applications, or games as they will consume significant bandwidth. Make sure that no one else in the household is downloading a large amount of data at the same time.

Conferencing Etiquette

You need a quiet, private room where you will be undisturbed for the duration of your interview. If required, book a conference room at your hospital or university. Prior to joining the virtual interview room, you will be joining the holding room, and this is your opportunity for a final check

DOI: 10.1201/9781003350422-9

of your video and audio transmission. Dress professionally for the occasion, just as you would for an in-person interview. You can keep a glass of water nearby but avoid drinking anything else. Canned drinks should be avoided as they can be misinterpreted as alcoholic beverages. Do not eat or chew gum during the interview.

Lighting

Choose a well-lit room, preferably with a light source behind the screen/monitor and behind the camera. This light source should ideally be white and preferably cold so as to not make you sweat. A white natural light LED bulb is perfect for this.

Avoid having the light source behind you as you will present your silhouette to the panellists. Having the light source on one side of you will create shadows on the opposite half of your face. This will make it hard for interviewers to see your expressions and may be distracting.

Background

A plain white or off-white background is the perfect backdrop for the video interview. Failing that, choose a wall with a neutral colour. Avoid having a window or any strong colours that may distract from you or, even worse, colours that may blend you into the background.

Avoid having a busy background, especially with pictures, paintings, or bookshelves. If you want to add some colour, then a simple houseplant will do. If you are adding props, be mindful of how the picture is framed; you do not want plants sticking out of your head!

Be aware that colours may come through differently on camera. This is especially the case on lower-quality webcams, such as those built into laptops. Some webcams may not have a wide colour range and suffer from poor colour reproduction. Therefore, it is worth checking with a preview on whichever application you are using to make sure that you can be seen clearly. Lighting can also have a big effect on colour representation on camera, so it is worth ensuring that lighting is set up beforehand.

Equipment

Whilst it is not necessary to have audio-visual equipment that would rival the BBC, investing in a good-quality webcam and having a clear mic available will serve you well beyond just the interview.

Laptop webcams are what most people are going to use. If you are using one, you must make sure the lighting is adequate as these webcams typically have the smallest of sensors. These sensors struggle in low-light conditions and the subsequent software correction can result in poor image quality and colour reproduction. A dedicated webcam usually results in a much-improved picture quality and can be used in future presentations and conferencing. These devices can come with additional features, such as superior image processing and adjustable field of view, as well as privacy features. With the sky being the limit, it is important not to get too carried away. Typically, a 1080p or 2K webcam with good low-light performance should suffice. Adjustable field of view is a bonus as it allows you to frame yourself perfectly in the resultant video output.

Choosing a good microphone is important so that the interviewers can hear your voice clearly and without unwanted interference. Whilst software noise cancelling has improved dramatically in recent years, having high-quality input will ensure that your voice will sound as natural as possible without any unwanted cut-outs and noise. Using earphones with a clip-on mic attachment is a perfectly adequate option that will sound better than a standard laptop-embedded mic. A dedicated headset is a better option but try and find one that is not too bulky or horribly oversized. Alternatively, a dedicated mic on a stand is a good if not slightly overkill option, but it has the advantage of being more versatile if you were to use it in future projects or video lectures. If you do go down the dedicated mic route, choose one that has good software support with a USB connection and an auto-levelling function. Companies like RØDE, Marantz, and Shure all produce consumer and prosumer mics for this purpose.

Camera Positioning

The ideal camera position is as close as possible to eye level, directly in front of you. Ideally, you should be looking into the camera whilst answering questions but still have the video feed in your peripheral vision so that you can respond to visual cues and mirror body language.

It is best to avoid having the camera positioned too high that you have to look up and also has the effect of making to appear smaller than you are. Position it too low and you might give panellists a good view up your nose and make it difficult for them to read your facial expressions.

Microphone Positioning

The ideal position of the microphone depends on which one you intend to use. If you are using a built-in mic on a laptop or a tablet, you have little choice in this matter. However, there are things you can do to improve the quality of your audio transmission. Make sure that the mic opening is not blocked with debris. Gently blow or clean the opening, taking care not to damage the mic inside. If you must, use compressed air, then hold it at least eight inches away to ensure that the pressure from the can does not damage the diaphragm of the mic. These mics are also incredibly sensitive, so avoid placing anything (e.g. paper, flashcards) on them as they will pick up the rustle if you move them during the interview.

If you are using a clip-on mic, it is best clipped between the top buttons of a shirt or anywhere on your clothing where it is not likely to rustle against your clothing as you talk.

A headset mic is best adjusted close to your mouth and away from your nose so that it does not pick up breath sounds.

A dedicated dynamic mic or condenser mic should be either on a table stand or on an adjustable boom. It is possible to keep the mic out of view by keeping it either above or below you and out of the frame of the camera. These mics are designed to pick up voices and have excellent sound isolation characteristics. They work best when pointed at you and typically can be adjusted to either a near or far setting depending on your setup.

Seating Position

Adjusting your seating so that you are close as possible to eye level with the camera is important for the reasons discussed earlier. Furthermore, it is important to consider what tics and movements you are likely to do when answering questions. Ideally, you need to sit upright and comfortably. If you are someone who is likely to swivel or rock in the chair when stressed or answering questions, it is important to have a chair without those functions as it will be very distracting to the panellists.

Application Settings

When setting up the video-conferencing application, make sure you have an account with your work or NHS email. If you have a profile picture, make sure it is appropriate for the occasion. Take time to go through your video and audio settings to make sure that the video is clear, focused, and appropriately zoomed in. Where available, hardware acceleration should be turned on, and depending on the type of mic and the level of background noise, you can adjust noise suppression settings to get a clear natural audio transmission. If you are unsure, these settings are best left on auto.

chapter nine

Clinical Scenarios

**William Rea, Sharukh Jamal Zuberi, Muhammad Salik,
Gopikanthan Manoharan, Gargi Pandey, Goran Ameer
Ahmed, Joshua Gaetos, Anokha Oomman Joseph, and
Janso Padickakudi Joseph**

General Surgery

Clinical Scenario 1: Post-Operative Desaturation

You are asked to see a 59-year-old gentleman on the ward, day 4 post-laparotomy for ischaemic bowel. He has a saturation of 84% on 2 litres of oxygen and a respiratory rate of 30. How would you approach this patient?

Based on the information provided, I am concerned about a potential post-operative respiratory complication, with pulmonary embolism or a respiratory tract infection following major surgery being my primary differentials. I would attend to this patient immediately and ask the nurse to call the outreach team.

I would assess the patient in a systematic way based on the CCrISP principles. In view of the recent pandemic, I would make sure I take relevant PPE precautions. I would talk to the patient to ensure the patency of his airway. I would put him on 15 litres of high-flow oxygen via a non-rebreather mask with a reservoir bag and attach him to a pulse oximeter. I would initially aim for a saturation of 92% and above. If the patient is verbally responsive, I would move on to assessing breathing and start with adequate exposure. If not, he would require airway adjuncts.

I would inspect for central cyanosis, bilateral chest movement, use of any accessory muscles, and any intercostal recessions and look for any distended neck veins. I would palpate to confirm the tracheal position and percuss the thorax to look for any hyper-resonance or dullness. I would auscultate the chest anteriorly and posteriorly in a sitting position to ascertain air entry and breath sounds. I would also listen to the heart sounds. Simultaneously, I would keep an eye on the pulse oximeter to see saturation on 15 litres of high-flow oxygen. I would check the patient's latest COVID-19 swab status. I recognise at this point that this patient needs an ABG and a chest x-ray.

DOI: 10.1201/9781003350422-10

I would move on to circulation to complete the assessment. I would check the central and peripheral capillary refill, feel the extremities, and ask for the patient's blood pressure and pulse rate. As this is a post-op inpatient, he might already have a Foley catheter, and I would ask for hourly output in the last 24 hours. I would ensure this patient has peripheral venous access in the form of two large-bore IV cannulas. I would draw blood and send for a full blood count, urea and electrolytes, liver function test, c-reactive protein, bone profile, and blood cultures if the patient is febrile. I would request an ECG. If the patient has tachyarrhythmia, this might require specialist management.

As part of disability, I would then calculate the patient's GCS and check the blood glucose and temperature. Following that, I would expose and examine the patient's abdomen, including the removal of any dressings to carefully inspect the wound and examine his calves.

I would go through this patient's medical history to see if he has any background of, for example, COPD, asthma, congestive cardiac failure, or any other cardiorespiratory pathologies. I would read the op-note to see the findings and specifics of the procedure done four days ago and whether any specific instructions were given. I would go through the patient's medication chart to see if he is on any bronchodilators/steroid inhalers and if he has had his relevant thromboembolic prophylaxis prescribed and administered, and I would see if he is on any other relevant medications. I would see the latest ward round notes to see if there were any specific concerns. I would calculate the Wells score.

With all this information, I would escalate to my registrar and potentially the consultant surgeon. I might require the help of the medical outreach team as the patient might be having a life-threatening pathology and might require a higher level of care. I might need to call the ITU team. During this situation, I would delegate some tasks, such as running the ABG, to my FY1. Based on the patient's initial response to treatment and assessment, he might need a CTPA to exclude a pulmonary embolus. If this were my top differential, I would start therapeutic anticoagulation with low-molecular-weight heparin. Alternatively, if the patient is septic and I suspect hospital-acquired pneumonia, I would start sepsis 6 and antibiotics. If there is any concern over the patient's abdominal examination, I would include a CT for the abdomen/pelvis.

I would be mindful of the distress the patient is in and would update him as much as practically possible and involve family or next of kin at an appropriate time.

- Probes
  - What are your immediate concerns?
  - What information would you gather while assessing the patient?

- What investigations would you consider in such a patient?
- How would you escalate this patient?
- Positive markers
  - Appreciates the urgency of the situation and attends to the patient immediately
  - Assesses using a structured approach based on CCrISP principles
  - Keeps reassessing after intervening
  - Is mindful of the current pandemic situation
  - Requests initial investigations, including a CXR and ABG
  - Escalates appropriately (e.g. outreach, registrar)
  - Goes through relevant PMH/operation notes/medications
- Negative markers
  - Does not attend immediately
  - Uses an unstructured approach
  - Does not get appropriate investigations, such as ABG/CXR
  - Does not see the response to intervention
  - Fails to escalate to outreach and registrar

Clinical Scenario 2: Upper GI Bleed

You are the core surgical trainee on-call at a district teaching hospital. You are asked to see a 76-year-old alcoholic gentleman on the gastroenterology ward with haematemesis. He is hypotensive and tachycardic. How would you approach this patient?

I am concerned this patient is in hypovolaemic (haemorrhagic) shock owing to an upper gastrointestinal bleed secondary to oesophageal varices. My priorities would be to resuscitate, evaluate, and escalate appropriately. I would attend to this patient immediately and ask for an updated set of observations. If concerned about the vitals, I would request the ward team to put out a medical emergency call. I would also escalate this to my registrar early. This patient might require an emergency therapeutic endoscopy.

I would approach the assessment and management of the patient according to the CCrISP protocol. I would start with an A–E assessment. I would assess his airway by speaking to him and by looking and listening for any additional airway sounds signalling airway obstruction or bodily fluids in the oropharynx. If the patient is speaking, that indicates a patent airway, in which case I would move on. However, if there are abnormal airway sounds, I would use the wall-mounted suction to remove any liquid obstruction and insert an airway adjunct if required (either an oropharyngeal or nasopharyngeal airway).

I would then move on to assess his breathing, looking for any signs of respiratory distress or cyanosis. I would feel for his chest expansion and would listen to his lung fields for any abnormal breath sounds. I would request to know his respiratory rate and oxygen saturation. If the patient is hypoxic or tachypnoeic, I would request a chest x-ray and arterial blood gas analysis, as well as ensuring high-flow oxygen administration to maximise oxygen absorption and delivery.

Assessing his circulation, I would look for signs of shock by looking for pallor, clamminess, and decreased consciousness level, which could indicate poor perfusion of the tissues. I would also feel for a central and peripheral pulse to determine its presence, character, volume, rate, and rhythm. I would auscultate the precordium to assess the presence of any diminished or additional heart sounds. I would measure the patient's capillary refill time centrally, blood pressure, and heart rate. I might request an ECG if I am concerned about an arrhythmia.

The patient would require two large-bore IV cannulas, as well as having a set of baseline blood specimens for full blood count, urea and electrolytes, liver function tests, clotting, and two group and save samples for cross-matching. If an ABG was not performed earlier, a VBG should be taken at this point to assess the haemoglobin and lactate levels.

I would then assess his neurological function by calculating his Glasgow coma score (GCS) and requesting a blood glucose measurement. Finally, I would expose the patient, examine his abdomen, and perform a PR examination to look for any melaena.

I would also look at the patient's notes to find out about his medical history, in particular whether he is known to have oesophageal varices, given the history of alcohol abuse. Another differential is a bleeding peptic ulcer or malignancy. I would also want to see his drug chart to ensure he is not on any blood-thinning agents.

If my assessment confirms haemorrhagic shock secondary to an upper gastrointestinal bleed, my clinical priorities would be to ensure ongoing tissue perfusion, arranging a place of safety, and arranging therapeutic intervention.

I would resuscitate with blood transfusion, initially O-negative packed red blood cells, followed by type-specific cross-matched blood and possibly other blood products if indicated. I would activate the massive transfusion protocol.

At this stage, I am also considering my clinical team. If I have any FY1, I might delegate some tasks, including running the ABG or liaising with blood transfusion services to them. I hope my registrar has become available to assist with the care of this patient. A senior decision-maker is required at this stage, so if my registrar is not reachable, I would escalate this directly to my consultant. Therapeutic intervention with an oesophagogastroduodenoscopy (OGD) is indicated urgently if the patient does not respond to the resuscitation and continues to have ongoing upper GI bleeding. This patient should ideally be moved to a high-dependency unit or intensive care unit bed with the capability of invasive blood pressure monitoring.

In order to facilitate this, I would liaise with the blood transfusion laboratory, haematologist on-call, intensive care doctor, outreach team, and gastroenterologist on-call. This patient might possibly require a general anaesthetic to facilitate the OGD, so after discussion with the gastroenterologist, a call to the theatre coordinator and anaesthetist on-call might also be needed.

The patient and his family must be kept informed at all times, and I would keep the patient at the centre of care. The ward staff might also need some support after a very visual and emotive event, and I would explore if they were interested in a debriefing exercise after the event.

- Probes
  - What are your priorities?
  - What is your differential diagnosis?
  - What other information would you gather?
  - Who will be required to aid with the management of this patient?
- Positive markers
  - Attends to the patient immediately
  - Performs A–E assessment along with a clinical note and chart review
  - Recognises patient is in hypovolaemic shock and manages appropriately
  - Performs appropriate, timely escalation
- Negative markers
  - Fails to recognise a critically unwell patient
  - Passes responsibility to the medical team
  - Uses an unstructured approach to patient assessment

Clinical Scenario 3: Pancreatitis

You are the core surgical trainee on-call at a district general hospital. You are asked to see a 43-year-old patient in A&E with acute abdominal pain. Their amylase is 4000. You note they have a medical history of diabetes. How would you approach this patient?

Given the history and amylase value, this patient almost certainly has acute pancreatitis. I would attend to the patient urgently. My priority is to exclude systemic complications of acute pancreatitis, such as acute kidney injury, ARDS, and multi-organ failure. The patient would require admission to hospital, and I would consider what level of care they require.

I would do a quick A–E assessment using the CCrISP principles. If the patient is haemodynamically stable, I would take a history, with specific questions to establish the underlying cause of their pancreatitis. I would specifically ask about a history of gallstones and alcohol use. I would also assess their medical history, their regular medications (including any new medications), and their allergies. I would then examine the patient, performing respiratory, cardiovascular, and abdominal examinations. The respiratory examination would be looking for any evidence of pleural effusion or acute respiratory distress syndrome. The cardiovascular examination would be looking for evidence of intravascular depletion or dehydration. And the abdominal examination would be assessing for jaundice or evidence of retroperitoneal haemorrhage.

I would then review all available blood results and any relevant previous investigations. I want to see an FBC, U&E, LFTs, CRP, clotting, amylase/lipase, and an ABG. I would determine the Glasgow-Imrie score. If I am concerned about complicated pancreatitis, I would arrange a CT scan to determine if there is any necrosis or peripancreatic collections. If there are no previously conducted ultrasound scans, I would request this to exclude gallstones. If there is jaundice present, the patient might require an MRCP or ERCP.

Once I have assessed the patient, I would make use of the full team. I might delegate some tasks to the FY1 – for example, calculating the Glasgow-Imrie score. I would alert my registrar and inform them about my assessment and management of the patient. If the patient is sick, with multi-organ involvement, I would involve my registrar early.

In terms of management, the patient would need a strict fluid input and output chart with urinary catheterisation. The patient could continue oral intake but might need supplementation with aggressive IV fluids. I would not start antibiotics unless there was a clear source of infection as pancreatitis with cholangitis. Given this patient's history of diabetes, close monitoring of blood sugars is indicated. The patient could continue their regular diabetic medication. However, depending on how much oral intake they are able to tolerate, their blood glucose levels are likely to be variable. A variable rate insulin infusion (a sliding scale) might be required if the blood sugar levels are abnormal. The patient would also require a drug chart with their regular medications, analgesia, a VTE risk assessment with low-molecular-weight heparin, and anti-embolic stockings prescribed. They might also require antiemetics, antispasmodics, and PPIs in the PRN section.

If the patient had an acute kidney injury or had signs of ARDS, I would contact the outreach team and speak to the ITU registrar for consideration of this patient to be managed in a level 2 setting like HDU. If the patient had necrotising pancreatitis CT and associated conditions causing organ failure, I would discuss this patient with the local HPB team on-call.

At all times, I would keep the patient at the centre of care. I would explain the need for multiple investigations and the seriousness of their condition to them. If the patient had gallstone pancreatitis in particular, I would use visual aids to explain this to them.

- Probes
  - What is the likely diagnosis?
  - What are the most common causes of pancreatitis?
  - What would your priorities be during the assessment of the patient?
  - How would you assess severity of pancreatitis?
- Positive markers
  - Has a systematic approach to patient assessment
  - Considers complications of pancreatitis
  - Orders appropriate investigations
  - Escalates to the registrar and consultant appropriately
- Negative markers
  - Prescribes simple analgesia only
  - Does not consider the aetiology of pancreatitis
  - Does not consider possible complications of pancreatitis
  - Does not escalate appropriately
  - Does not consider a higher level of care

Clinical Scenario 4: Post-Operative Fever

You are the core surgical trainee on colorectal surgery. You see a 37-year-old gentleman on the ward round. He is two days post–right hemicolectomy for malignancy. He has a temperature of 38.1°C. How would you approach this patient?

In a patient with a low-grade fever post-operatively, I would be concerned about an infection. The most significant source of this is an anastomotic leak. However, given that patient is only day 2 post-op, I would also be considering other sources of infection, such as intra-abdominal collection, chest infection, urinary tract infection, and skin infection of the operative wound. I would also consider DVT/PE as a non-infective source of post-op fever.

I would review the patient's observations and most recent blood tests, as well as the operation note and anaesthetic chart. I would also make note of the patient's comorbidities, particularly issues that could contribute to immunosuppression or wound breakdown, such as diabetes or taking steroids.

I would assess this patient according to the CCrISP protocol. I would ensure his airway is patent and self-maintained. I would then look at his breathing, feel for any asymmetrical chest movement or crepitus in the chest wall, auscultate the chest for any abnormal breath sounds, and measure the respiratory rate and oxygen saturation levels. If he is hypoxic or tachypnoeic, then I would start oxygen supplementation.

I would then move to assess his circulation, looking for any signs of hypotension or impaired perfusion. I would feel for his central and peripheral pulses for rate, rhythm, character, and volume. I would auscultate the precordium for abnormal heart sounds and then measure his heart rate, blood pressure, capillary refill time, and temperature.

I would cannulate the patient and send off a full set of blood specimens. I would then assess his consciousness using the Glasgow coma scale and request a blood glucose measurement.

I would fully expose the patient and examine him to attempt to determine the source of the infection. Given the patient's history, there are multiple possible sources: respiratory, urinary, skin (either cellulitis, phlebitis, or surgical incision), or intra-abdominal. I would take down any dressings to inspect the wounds, review drain content and volume, and palpate the abdomen to determine any evidence of peritonism suggesting an intra-abdominal source. The patient is likely to be catheterised, so a urine dip is likely to be positive, so I would ask the nursing team to send off a sample for culture and sensitivity. I would also examine the calves to ensure there is no DVT. I would also look at any peripheral or central lines.

A chest x-ray would be indicated if a respiratory source is suspected. Though an anastomotic leak on day 2 is unusual, it remains the most concerning source of infection. If I was concerned about an anastomotic leak, I would request a CT scan to confirm this. If I suspect a DVT, I would calculate a Wells score and obtain a venous Doppler. If I found an infected line, I would remove it.

I would also review the patient's drug chart and see if he is on immunosuppressants or antibiotics. I would also look at the operative note to see if there was any complication during the surgery.

Following my assessment and management plan, I would then contact the responsible registrar or consultant and present the patient to them with a summary of what treatments and investigations I have initiated. I would ask my FY1 to help with documentation and make sure the blood work is drawn.

If the CT revealed an anastomotic leak, then the patient would require a return to theatre to take down the anastomosis, wash out the abdomen, and most likely form a stoma as a second anastomosis would be at an unacceptably high risk of breakdown.

- Probes
  - What are the causes of post-op fever?
  - How would you investigate the source of infection?
  - What are the non-infective causes of fever?
- Positive markers
  - Uses a systematic assessment
  - Considers the sources of infection
  - Considers investigative methods
- Negative markers
  - Fixates on anastomotic leak
  - Does not consider different causes of post-operative fever

Clinical Scenario 5: Wound Dehiscence

You are the core surgical trainee on general surgery. On the ward round you see 55-year-old gentleman, day 5 post–emergency laparotomy, for perforated diverticular disease. The patient is complaining of discomfort in the abdomen, and there is copious pink fluid discharging from the wound.

In this scenario, given the post-operative timing, the pink fluid makes me concerned the patient is at risk of wound dehiscence resulting in a burst abdomen. Other differentials include wound infection or infected seroma.

I would assess this patient according to the CCRISP protocol. I would ensure the patient was speaking to me and had a patent airway.

I would then look at his breathing, feel for any asymmetrical chest movement, auscultate for any abnormal breath sounds, and measure the respiratory rate and oxygen saturation levels. If he is hypoxic or tachypnoeic, I would then request the nursing staff to administer oxygen.

Then I would move to assess his circulation, looking for any signs of hypotension or impaired perfusion. I would feel for his central and peripheral pulses for rate, rhythm, character, and volume. I would auscultate the precordium for abnormal heart sounds and then measure his heart rate, blood pressure, capillary refill time, and temperature. If he is hypotensive, I would administer a fluid bolus of crystalloid, after which I would reassess to see if there had been any improvement.

If he is tachycardic, I would request an ECG to rule out tachyarrhythmia. If he is febrile, then he would need blood cultures and antibiotic administration. The presence of fever makes the diagnosis of infection highly likely, given the patient's history, and should trigger the initiation of the sepsis 6 bundle.

I would then assess his consciousness using the Glasgow coma scale, and also request a blood glucose measurement.

I would then examine the abdomen more closely. I would take down the abdominal dressing and inspect the laparotomy wound, looking for surrounding erythema, induration, swelling, fluctuance, necrosis, tenderness, crepitus, and discharge.

If there is discharge, I would note the volume and character of discharge – is it serous, purulent, or bloody? If the discharge is coming from the laparotomy wound with no other signs of infection, I would be concerned that this patient is about to have a wound dehiscence resulting in a burst abdomen, which could be very alarming for the patient and the staff.

If abdominal wound dehiscence is already present, I would cover the wound with warm saline-soaked swabs after pushing the back bowel into the abdomen. I would have more saline swabs ready at the bedside. I would escalate this to my registrar immediately. I would involve the ward sister so that I have an extra pair of hands with me. I would also contact the anaesthetic team and the theatre coordinator and book the patient and acquire consent from him for an urgent return to theatre for closure of the laparotomy wound.

Alternatively, if I found that this patient has a seroma or wound infection, I might take out some stitches or staples and start antibiotics.

- Probes
  - What is your differential diagnosis?
  - What are your priorities?
  - What other information would you gather?
  - Who else would you like to involve in this patient's care?
- Positive markers
  - Considers malignancy as the most likely diagnosis
  - Constructs a reasonable differential diagnosis
  - Requests appropriate investigations
  - Escalates to the registrar or consultant appropriately
  - Has a structured approach to patient assessment
  - Recognises that the pink fluid is the classic sign seen before a burst abdomen
- Negative markers
  - Uses an unstructured approach to patient assessment
  - Does not involve the wider healthcare team
  - Does not consider differentials more serious than a wound infection
  - Does not escalate

Clinical Scenario 6: Trauma

You are asked to see a 29-year-old patient following a road traffic accident. He had to be extracted from the car. He seems to be in significant pain and is clutching his abdomen. How would you approach this patient?

I am concerned that this patient has significant intra-abdominal injuries following the road traffic accident. This could be due to a viscus perforation or internal bleeding. Depending on the patient's haemodynamic stability, he might require a scan or might need to go directly to theatre.

I would attend to this patient immediately after putting out a trauma call. I would approach the patient using an ATLS approach. I would ensure the patient's c-spine is secured with three-point immobilisation. I would assess the airway by first speaking to him. I would ensure high-flow oxygen is being administered. If he verbally responds, indicating a patent and self-maintained airway, I would move on to assess his breathing.

I would look for bilateral chest rising, bilateral chest sounds, and a central trachea. I would palpate for chest wall tenderness and surgical emphysema and auscultate the chest for breath sounds in all regions. I would then measure the oxygen saturation and respiratory rate.

If the airway is intact, I would then move on to circulation and haemorrhage. I would assess the patient's heart rate, blood pressure, and capillary refill time. I would inspect and palpate the patient's abdomen, then look for symmetry of the ASIS bilaterally and palpate the long bones. I am doing this in C because I am looking for a source of bleeding. I would also look around the patient for any evidence of external haemorrhage.

I would ensure that bilateral large-bore access is gained. At the same time, I would take blood specimens for venous blood gas, FBC, U&E, LFTs, and cross-match. If the patient is hypotensive and tachycardic, he might benefit from a blood transfusion. If there is an ultrasound-trained member of the trauma team present, a FAST scan could be used to determine the presence of intra-abdominal fluid.

For disability, I would calculate his GCS and assess for pupillary reaction to light. I would then expose the patient, fully examine him, perform a log roll, and digital rectal examination.

As I am concerned that this patient has significant intra-abdominal injuries, I would be quick to escalate this to my registrar and consultant. The anaesthetic team should already be in attendance as part of the trauma team.

Depending on the patient's response to initial resuscitation and the results of his FAST scan, we might decide to perform a CT for the abdomen and pelvis if he is stable. Alternatively, we might have to go directly to theatres for an exploratory trauma laparotomy if the patient is unstable.

This decision-making requires communication with A&E, nursing staff, radiology, blood transfusion, and theatre teams. Given the urgency of the situation, a second CEPOD theatre might need to be opened up.

I appreciate that this is a stressful time for the patient. I would keep him at the centre of care. I would explain what is happening to him in a timely manner. I would ensure that he has adequate analgesia. If he could consent to surgery, then I would do this. However, in this trauma situation, he might require a consent form 4. I would update his next of kin.

- Probes
  - What is your differential diagnosis?
  - What are your priorities?
  - What other information would you gather?
  - Who else would you like to involve in this patient's care?
- Positive markers
  - Understands ATLS structure
  - Takes a multidisciplinary approach to the trauma patient
  - Knows when not to consider a CT
  - Escalates appropriately
- Negative markers
  - Performs an unstructured examination
  - Does not escalate
  - Fails to involve other members of the trauma team
  - Wants a CT in an unstable patient

Clinical Scenario 7: C. difficile *Infection*

You are the core surgical trainee. You are asked to see a 65-year-old lady who has been treated for diverticulitis with several courses of antibiotics. She now presents with abdominal pain and diarrhoea. How would you approach this patient?

I am concerned this patient has *C. difficile* colitis secondary to overgrowth following repeated antibiotic courses. My other differentials include diverticulitis or complications of diverticulitis, such as a diverticular perforation or abscess.

Given the history of diarrhoea, the patient should be seen in a side room with the required isolation precautions. I would approach her using a CCrISP approach. I would take a full history, enquiring about her abdominal pain and taking note of what antibiotic she has received, in how many courses, and in what time frame.

I would also ask about the patient's diverticular disease, how often she gets flares, if she has had any investigations, and if she has had any complications from her diverticulitis. I would ask about her medical history and drug history, including allergies. I would also ask if this patient has ever had a colonoscopy and, if so, how long ago.

I would then examine this patient. If I feel the patient is extremely unwell, I would use an A–E approach.

Speaking to the patient and receiving a response would ensure her airway is patent and self-maintained. I would then look at her breathing, feel for any asymmetrical chest movement, auscultate the chest for any abnormal breath sounds, and measure the respiratory rate and oxygen saturation levels. If she is hypoxic or tachypnoeic, I would then request the clinic staff to locate an oxygen cylinder to administer oxygen.

Then I would move to assess the patient's circulation, looking for any signs of hypotension or impaired perfusion. I would feel for her central and peripheral pulses for rate, rhythm, character, and volume. I would auscultate the precordium for abnormal heart sounds and then measure her heart rate, blood pressure, capillary refill time, and temperature.

If the patient is hypotensive, I would administer a fluid bolus of crystalloid, after which I would reassess to see if there had been any improvement. If she is tachycardic, I would request an ECG to rule out tachyarrhythmia. If she is febrile, then she would need blood cultures and antibiotic administration.

I would then assess the patient's consciousness using the Glasgow coma scale and also request a blood glucose measurement.

I would then assess the abdomen more closely. I would inspect, palpate, percuss, and auscultate the abdomen to determine the location of pain, its severity, and the presence of any peritoneal irritation.

Following history taking and examination, I would review any investigations available and review any notes available – either from this admission or previous documentation. My priority with the assessment would be to exclude an acute abdomen.

I would send for blood tests, including FBC, U&E, LFTs, CRP, and group and save. If I am clinically concerned about *C. difficile* colitis, then I would ask for a stool sample to be sent to microbiology for toxin gene (PCR) and glutamate dehydrogenase EIA (GDH). If this is positive, then we would need to do a toxin enzyme immunoassay (EIA). If this also comes back as positive, then the patient likely has *C. difficile*, and this needs mandatory reporting. Trust policy on isolation, enhanced nursing care, and cleaning protocol would need to be followed.

If I am concerned about the complication of diverticular disease, such as a perforation or abscess, then I would obtain a CT for the abdomen/pelvis.

Depending on the severity of the *C. difficile* colitis, if it is a moderately severe disease, I would commence oral metronidazole, and if it is a very severe disease, the patient would need IV vancomycin per the trust protocol. I would speak to my registrar about the patient's case. In particular, I would enquire about where the patient should be admitted to – medicine or surgery. I would speak to nursing and bed management to facilitate admission.

I would keep the patient at the centre of care at all times, communicating my findings and planning with her. Given her recurrent episodes of diverticulitis, we might also need to consider a long-term plan for her in terms of surgical resection. I would ensure that this patient has an appropriate follow-up in the colorectal clinic to discuss this.

- Probes
  - What is your differential diagnosis?
  - What are your priorities?
  - What other information would you gather?
  - Who else would you like to involve in this patient's care?
- Positive markers
  - Considers more than one differential
  - Approaches the case in a systematic manner
  - Escalates appropriately
- Negative markers
  - Uses an unstructured approach
  - Focuses on a single diagnosis
  - Ignores or fails to take into account previous attacks of diverticulitis

Clinical Scenario 8: Post-Operative Breast Haematoma

You are asked to see a 54-year-old on the general surgery ward, day 2 post-mastectomy. The patient has 300 ml of blood in her drain. She is on apixaban, which was restarted earlier today. How would you approach this patient?

I would review the patient immediately. I am concerned the patient is bleeding from her mastectomy wound. She might require a return to theatre.

I would initially assess using the CCrISP algorithm. I would make sure patient's airway and breathing are intact by talking to the patient. I would check patient's observations and haemodynamic state by measuring oxygen saturation, heart rate, blood pressure, and capillary refill. I would make sure the patient has two large-bore IV lines.

I would give patient high-flow oxygen initially. If the patient is hypotensive and tachycardic I would start 20 ml/kg warm crystalloids stat. I would take an ABG to check for lactate, Hb and base deficit. I would also take blood for G&S, FBC, U&E, clotting, and LFTs.

Depending on the shock state, if she is in stage 3 or 4 haemorrhagic shock, I would activate the major haemorrhage protocol.

I would expose the patient to examine her wound for evidence of haematoma, such as bruising and tense swelling of the mastectomy site. I would examine the drain content.

I would review the notes, in particular the operative note. I would see if there were any concerns over haemostasis.

If there is evidence of active bleeding, I would call my registrar and inform the consultant in charge of the patient because she might need to go back to theatre to control bleeding. At this stage, I do not think there is a role for additional investigations, such as an ultrasound scan of the breast.

In the meantime, although there is no direct reversal agent for apixaban, I would call the haematologist on-call to discuss the case and determine the need for plasma or prothrombin complex concentrate (Beriplex). While seniors are on the way, I would apply a pressure dressing to tamponade any active bleeding. I would alert the anaesthetic team, theatres, and nursing staff that this patient needs to go back to theatre urgently.

I would explain the situation to the patient and provide her with analgesia and reassurance. I would prepare the consent forms for my registrar. I would update the next of kin and document in the notes.

- Probes
  - What are your priorities?
  - What other information would you gather?
  - What investigations would you do?
  - How would you escalate this patient's care?
- Positive markers
  - Recognises that the patient is actively bleeding and this is a surgical emergency
  - Recognises that this requires a team-based approach
  - Assesses the patient with a structured A–E approach
  - Requests appropriate investigations (e.g. group and screen, FBC, coagulation panel) and anticipates the need for immediate blood transfusion and correcting pre-existing coagulopathy
  - Escalates to the registrar or consultant appropriately
- Negative markers
  - Does not attend immediately and recognise the situation as a surgical emergency
  - Fails to include other members of the surgical team (anaesthetists, theatre nurses, etc.)
  - Uses an unstructured approach to patient assessment
  - Does not anticipate the need for immediate blood transfusion and correcting pre-existing coagulopathy
  - Does not escalate patient care appropriately

Clinical Scenario 9: Inflammatory Bowel Disease

You are asked to see a 38-year-old gentleman on the gastroenterology ward with inflammatory bowel disease who is complaining of abdominal pain. He has been on steroids for ten days for treatment of a flare. How would you approach this patient?

I would attend to this patient as soon as possible. As I am on my way to see the patient, I would think of the differential diagnoses of bowel perforation, toxic megacolon, and acute severe (fulminant) colitis. The patient might require operative intervention.

I would assess the patient using the CCrISP algorithm. I would make sure the airway and breathing are intact by checking to the patient is able to talk and checking breath sounds, respiratory rate, and oxygen saturation. I would check the circulatory status by checking heart rate, blood pressure, and urine output. I would make sure the patient has two widebore IV lines.

I would give high-flow oxygen to start with and start 20 ml/kg crystalloids stat. If I suspect sepsis, I would make sure the sepsis 6 bundle measures are carried out. I would give oxygen, IV antibiotics, and fluids, take specimens for lactate and blood culture, and measure the patient's urine output.

I would then examine the patient in general for signs of dehydration, pallor, and jaundice. I would examine the patient's abdomen to check for tenderness, distension, peritonism, scars, and hernial orifices. I would also check bowel sounds and do a PR exam to check for blood, mucus, and any rectal mass.

I would examine the patient's charts for observations, the fluid balance chart, and the Bristol stool chart for frequency and consistency of stool. I would also go through the patient's history and background medical issues. I would check the patient's latest blood tests paying, particular attention to WCC, CRP, and lactate levels. I would get a new set of blood and take an ABG.

I would keep the patient nil by mouth and arrange for an urgent CT AP with IV contrast.

At this stage, I would escalate to my registrar or consultant. I might need to discuss this with the on-call radiologist to make sure that they understand the urgency of the scan. I would liaise directly with the radiographers to make sure that the patient gets an early slot. I would also discuss the patient's care with the medical team to see if there are any treatment alternatives, such as escalation to biologics.

Depending on the assessment and CT findings, the patient might need ongoing conservative management or urgent surgery in the form of subtotal colectomy if the colitis is acutely severe. I would keep the patient at the centre of care, involving him in the decision-making. I would ensure that he has adequate analgesia and symptomatic control of nausea or fever. If the patient does have a perforation or flare of IBD unresponsive to medical management, he would need surgical intervention. After discussion with my seniors, I would prepare a consent form for the patient, inform the anaesthetic team and theatre coordinator, and book the patient for a laparotomy.

- Probes
  - What are your priorities?
  - What other information would you gather?
  - What investigations would you do?
  - How would you escalate this patient's care?
- Positive markers
  - Recognises that the patient has IBD unresponsive to medical therapy
  - Recognises that this requires a team-based approach
  - Assesses the patient with a structured A–E approach
  - Requests appropriate investigations, including CT scan
  - Escalates to the registrar or consultant appropriately
- Negative markers
  - Does not attend immediately and recognise the situation as a surgical emergency
  - Fails to include other members of the team (gastroenterologists, radiologists, theatre team, etc.)
  - Uses an unstructured approach to patient assessment
  - Does not escalate patient care appropriately

Clinical Scenario 10: Trauma

You are the core surgical trainee on trauma. You are asked to see a 25-year-old who presents to A&E with a penetrating knife injury to the right upper abdomen. How would you approach this patient?

I am concerned that this patient has intra-abdominal injuries following their knife injury. I would be specifically worried that there might be damage to the liver, gallbladder, hepatic triad, duodenum, head of pancreas, or IVC. However, I also need to consider the possibility of a trans-compartmental injury, with possible diaphragmatic injury causing a haemopneumothorax or haemopericardium.

I would attend to this patient immediately and would activate the trauma team. I would approach the patient using ATLS principles. I would ensure the patient's c-spine is secured with three-point immobilisation.

I would assess the airway by first speaking to them. I would ensure high-flow oxygen is being administered. If they verbally respond, indicating a patent and self-maintained airway, I would move on to assess their breathing. I would look for bilateral chest rising, bilateral chest sounds, and a central trachea. I would palpate for chest wall tenderness and surgical emphysema and auscultate the chest for breath sounds in all regions. I would then measure the oxygen saturation and respiratory rate.

If the airway is intact, I would then move on to circulation and haemorrhage. I would assess the patient's heart rate, blood pressure, and capillary refill time. I would inspect and palpate the patient's abdomen, look for symmetry of the ASIS bilaterally, then palpate the long bones. I would also look around the patient for any evidence of external haemorrhage.

I would ensure that bilateral large-bore access is gained. At the same time, I would take blood for venous blood gas, FBC, U&E, LFTs, and crossmatch. If the patient is hypotensive and tachycardic, I would transfuse blood.

If there is an ultrasound-trained member of the trauma team present, a FAST scan could be used to determine the presence of intra-abdominal fluid in Morrison's pouch. This would also assess for potential diaphragmatic injury if there were haemothorax or pneumothorax on the lung windows and also exclude a haemopericardium.

For disability, I would calculate the GCS and assess for pupillary reaction to light. As I am concerned that this patient has intra-abdominal injuries, I would be quick to escalate this to my registrar and consultant as they are likely to require a laparotomy.

Depending on the patient's response to initial resuscitation and the results of the FAST scan, we might decide to perform a CT scan or alternatively go directly to theatres for a laparotomy. This decision-making would require communication with A&E, nursing staff, radiology, blood transfusion, and theatre teams.

I would also ensure that I explain what is happening to the patient and liaise with the family.

- Probes
  - What are your concerns?
  - Who will need to be informed?
  - What investigations would you like to perform?
- Positive markers
  - Uses a systematic approach
  - Recognises the possibility of trans-compartmental injuries
  - Considers either scans or theatres, depending on how stable the patient is

- Negative markers
  - Uses an unstructured examination
  - Does not involve other specialities or colleagues

Clinical Scenario 11: Acute Cholecystitis

You are asked to see a 62-year-old gentleman on the ward with acute chole-cystitis. He has been on antibiotics for five days. He is complaining of severe abdominal pain over the last few hours and is now spiking a temperature.

In this scenario, I am concerned this patient has a complication from cho-lecystitis like gallbladder perforation, new onset cholangitis, or an unre-lated abdominal catastrophe like perforated DU.

I would examine the patient immediately as I am concerned he has sepsis. I would assess using the CCrISP algorithm. I would assess his air-way first by speaking to him. I would ensure he is on high-flow oxygen. If he responds, I would move on to assess his breathing. I would look for bilateral chest rising, bilateral chest sounds, and a central trachea. If his airway is intact, I would move on to circulation. I would assess the patient's heart rate, blood pressure, and capillary refill time. I would ensure that bilateral large-bore access is gained. I would take blood spec-imens for blood gas, FBC, U&E, LFTs, clotting profile, and cross-match. For disability, I would calculate his GCS and obtain a temperature and blood glucose. I would make sure the patient has adequate analgesia on board.

Given the scenario, I am concerned the patient has sepsis, and hence, I would initiate the sepsis 6 bundle. I would take blood cultures, measure lactate on the ABG, measure urine output, and give the patient oxygen, IV fluids, and IV antibiotics. I would also request a COVID-19 swab test.

If unstable, initially, I would start IV crystalloids at 20 ml/kg. I would give a second bolus if the patient is still hypotensive after the first one. I would be cautious with fluid resuscitation in a patient with a history of heart disease to avoid volume overload. I would aim to maintain his mean arterial pressure (MAP) equal and above 65, and if this is not achievable with fluids, I would contact ITU to assess the patient to con-sider vasopressors.

After initial assessment and management, I would review the patient's notes and check drug charts. I would let my registrar know, but I would arrange for an urgent CT abdomen and pelvis to get a definitive diagnosis. In the meantime, I would escalate to second-line antibiotics after checking trust microbiology guidelines and the patient's allergies.

Depending on the CT scan, the patient's ongoing management might include emergency surgical intervention if the patient has a perforated duodenal ulcer or a perforated gallbladder, or it might include emergency gallbladder drainage by interventional radiology if the patient has a gall-bladder empyema.

I would discuss this patient with the ITU registrar and transfer this patient to the high-dependency unit for more frequent monitoring and support. I would explain the scan findings and the plan to the patient.

- Probes
  - What is your diagnosis?
  - How would you manage this patient?
- Positive markers
  - Assesses the patient with a structured A–E approach
  - Requests appropriate investigations
  - Recognises the need for monitoring in HDU
- Negative markers
  - Uses an unstructured approach to patient assessment
  - Does not escalate appropriately

Clinical Scenario 12: Ectopic Pregnancy

You are the core surgical trainee. You see a 37-year-old Jehovah's Witness patient with right iliac fossa pain. She is haemodynamically unstable. How would you approach this patient?

In this scenario, I am concerned that the cause of the haemodynamic instability and right iliac fossa pain is either due to hypovolemic shock from a ruptured ectopic pregnancy or septic shock from a perforated appendix. The patient might also have had another abdominal catastrophe.

I would attend to this patient immediately. I would assess this patient using the CCrISP algorithm. First, I would speak to the patient and make sure her airway is intact. At the same time, I would give high-flow oxygen via a non-rebreather face mask. I would assess the adequacy of the patient's breathing by looking for chest expansion, checking for the tracheal position, listening to breath sounds, and oxygen saturation. At the same time, I would make sure two large IV lines are in place and she is working. I would do blood gas, FBC, U&E, LFTs, clotting profile, and cross-match.

I would check the patient's circulation by checking her heart rate, blood pressure, and capillary refill time. I would start with 1 litre (20 ml/kg) of warm crystalloids stat.

I would also perform a general and abdominal examination to establish a differential diagnosis. If the patient is showing signs of sepsis, like fever, warm peripheries, and flushed face, I would initiate the sepsis 6 bundle to manage her initially. This involves giving IV fluids to maintain a MAP of 65 or more, stat IV antibiotics, and high-flow oxygen. Before the antibiotics, I would take blood specimens for culture and sensitivity, and I would also check the patient's lactate and insert a urinary catheter to assess urine output.

If, however, on initial assessment, the patient is looking pale, tachycardic, hypotensive, and with prolonged capillary refill time, I would be concerned about internal bleeding and hypovolemic shock. I would escalate this to my registrar and consultant as this is a tricky situation, given the patient is a Jehovah's Witness. If stable enough after initial resuscitation, I would take a quick history and review medical notes. I would also check her capacity and check her beliefs regarding blood transfusion.

If not compos mentis, I would check for any documented advance decisions made by the patient. If any doubt about the validity of advance directives, I would act in the patient's best interest and start the transfusion. If the patient clearly has the capacity and refuses transfusion or has a valid advance decision stating refusal, I would explain the consequences of not having the blood transfusion. I would also check her beliefs regarding autologous transfusion and plan for a cell saver to be used in theatre if the patient goes on to have emergency surgery.

Depending on the results of tests and her initial response, the patient might need to have imaging or go to theatre immediately. I would liaise with the anaesthetist, the theatre coordinator, and the ITU registrar. If there are signs of ruptured ectopic pregnancy, like vaginal bleeding, positive pregnancy test, and haemorrhagic shock, I would alert the gynaecologists immediately.

I would make sure to document my management and discussion with the patient at the earliest possible chance.

- Probes
    - What is your differential diagnosis?
    - How would you manage this patient?
    - Would you transfuse blood?
- Positive markers
    - Assesses the patient with a structured A–E approach
    - Recognises patient is a Jehovah's Witness
    - Recognises the need to escalate early to the registrar and consultant
- Negative markers
    - Uses an unstructured approach to patient assessment
    - Does not involve other teams
    - Transfuses blood without considering the patient's wishes

Clinical Scenario 13: Bowel Obstruction

You are the core surgical trainee. A 56-year-old presents with a three-day history of vomiting and abdominal pain. He has a history of emergency laparotomy for an internal hernia. He is a type 2 diabetic on insulin.

In this scenario, I am concerned the patient has intestinal obstruction secondary to adhesions from his previous surgery. Other differentials include acute pancreatitis and diabetic ketoacidosis.

I would review the patient immediately. I would assess using the CCrISP algorithm. I would speak to the patient and make sure his airway is intact. At the same time, I would give high-flow oxygen via a non-rebreather face mask. I would assess the adequacy of the patient's breathing by looking for chest expansion, checking for the tracheal position, listening to breath sounds and oxygen saturation. I would assess the patient's heart rate, blood pressure and capillary refill time.

At the same time, I would make sure two large IV lines are inserted, and I would request an arterial blood gas, FBC, U&E, LFTs, amylase, and cross-match. I would check the patient's GCS and blood glucose levels.

I would expose and perform an abdominal examination. I would check for hydration, jaundice, abdominal distension, scars, peritonism, and bowel sounds. I would do a PR exam at the earliest convenience.

I would arrange for abdominal x-rays in the first instance. If this shows signs of bowel obstruction, I would make sure he is nursed at 45 degrees or more and ensure an NG tube is inserted as soon as possible to prevent aspiration of gastric contents. I would also insert a urinary catheter and check his urine output. I would ensure a fluid balance chart is followed by measuring all input and output. I would inform and escalate to my registrar once I have initiated a management plan.

Doing all this in a timely manner is labour-intensive, and according to the clinical urgency, I would need help from nursing staff and other members of the emergency team, like the outreach team and foundation doctors.

After initial assessment and management, I would get a CT scan of the abdomen and pelvis for a definitive diagnosis. If the obstruction is secondary to adhesions, the patient could be conservatively managed for up to 48 hours. However, if the obstruction does not resolve in this period, the patient would need to be taken to theatre for an emergency laparotomy and adhesiolysis.

I would update the patient and his family about his condition and document in the notes.

- Probes
  - What is your diagnosis?
  - How would you manage this patient?
  - Does this patient need to go to theatre?
- Positive markers
  - Applies appropriate management of bowel obstruction
  - Uses appropriate investigation
- Negative markers
  - Uses an unstructured approach to patient assessment
  - Does not consider a conservative approach initially

Clinical Scenario 14: Hernia

You are the core surgical trainee on-call at a central teaching hospital. You are asked to see a 75-year-old lady in A&E who has swelling in her groin, vomits, and has abdominal pain.

Given the patient's age and history, I am concerned this patient has an obstructed hernia; my priority would be to exclude a strangulated hernia. Given her gender, this is likely to be a femoral hernia; however, an obstructed inguinal hernia is the most likely diagnosis as it is the most common type of hernia.

I would attend to the patient urgently and do a quick A–E assessment using the CCrISP principles.

I would take a history, with specific questions to establish if the patient has an inguinal/femoral hernia. I would ask questions to establish if the hernia is just incarcerated or if there are symptoms to suggest obstruction and possibly ischaemia of the bowel within the hernia sac. I would ask about symptoms of bowel obstruction, such as abdominal pain, vomiting, failure to pass flatus, or open bowels.

I would ask about her medical history, medications, and allergies. I would examine the patient, performing an abdominal examination, looking to elicit any peritonism. I would then assess the swelling in the groin, firstly to establish if it is a hernia, and then to see if it is an inguinal or femoral hernia, and then to assess if it is incarcerated or strangulated.

I would then review all available blood results and any previous relevant investigations, such as a CT for the abdomen and pelvis or USS for the groin, to see if the patient has a hernia.

I would check if the patient's x-ray of the abdomen in A&E shows dilated small bowel loops suggesting an obstruction. I would check the lactate levels to assess if there are signs of ischaemia.

If the AXR confirms dilated small bowel loops, this suggests an obstructed hernia. The patient would need a nasogastric tube and IV fluids.

The patient would need to be nil by mouth. I would insert a catheter to monitor the urine output.

The patient needs to go to theatre for a repair of hernia +/− bowel resection +/− laparotomy. I would ensure that the patient gets an urgent senior surgical review by the on-call surgical registrar. I would then discuss this with the on-call anaesthetist and inform the theatre coordinator. I would speak to the bed manager to inform them of the admission.

I would explain the need for an operation to the patient and ask consent from her for theatre.

- Probes
  - What is the diagnosis?
  - Does this patient need a CT for the abdomen?
  - Can she be managed conservatively?
  - When will you plan for theatre?
- Positive markers
  - Uses A–E assessment along with previous imaging and chart review
  - Understands the importance of assessing if the patient has a strangulated hernia
  - Arranges appropriate investigations and plans for theatre
  - Appropriately escalates
- Negative markers
  - Fails to recognise the risk of a strangulated hernia
  - Does not work up the patient appropriately

Clinical Scenario 15: Anastomotic Leak

> You are the core surgical trainee on-call at a district general hospital. You are asked to prescribe a sleeping tablet for an agitated patient. The patient is a 67-year-old lady, day 5 post–laparoscopic anterior resection for rectal cancer.

Given the history, I am concerned this patient has an anastomotic leak, causing an infection that led to delirium. There could be other causes of sepsis, such as a chest infection or wound infection; however, given it has been five days since an anterior resection, my priority would be to exclude an anastomotic leak.

I would ask the ward nurse to do an urgent set of observations so that I have the most recent observations.

I would review the most recent blood tests, as well as the operation note and anaesthetic chart. I would also make note of the patient's comorbidities, particularly issues that could contribute to immunosuppression that might another factor in developing an anastomotic leak.

I would assess this patient according to the CCRISP protocol. I would ensure the airway is patent and self-maintained. I would then assess her breathing, feel for any asymmetrical chest movement, auscultate the chest for any abnormal breath sounds, and measure the respiratory rate and oxygen saturation levels. If she is hypoxic or tachypnoeic, then I would start oxygen supplementation.

I would then move to assess her circulation, looking for any signs of hypotension or impaired perfusion. I would feel for her central and peripheral pulses for rate, rhythm, character, and volume. I would auscultate the precordium for abnormal heart sounds and then measure her heart rate, blood pressure, capillary refill time, and temperature.

I would cannulate the patient and request for FBC, U&E, LFTs, amylase, clotting profile, and cross-match. I would also do blood gas and measure the lactate. I would then assess her consciousness using the Glasgow coma scale and request a blood glucose measurement.

I would fully expose the patient and examine her to attempt to determine the source of the infection. Given the patient's history, there are multiple possible sources: respiratory, urinary, wound, or intra-abdominal. I would inspect any dressings to inspect the wounds, review drain content and volume, and examine the abdomen to determine any evidence of peritonism suggesting an intra-abdominal source.

I would also review the patient's drug chart and see if he is on immunosuppressants or antibiotics. I would also look at the operative note to see if there was any complication during the surgery.

If there are signs of abdominal peritonism and the patient is stable, I would arrange a CT for the abdomen and pelvis after a discussion with my registrar.

If I was concerned about sepsis, I would initiate the sepsis 6 bundle and ensure that lactate, urine output monitoring, and blood cultures have been sent off. I would also ensure the patient is given IV fluids, IV antibiotics, and oxygen supplementation.

I would also request a urine dip for culture and sensitivity and order a chest x-ray to rule out other sources of infection. However, at day 5, an anastomotic leak is the most concerning source of infection.

Depending on the CT findings, the patient might likely need to be taken back to theatre for an emergency laparotomy and end colostomy. I would speak to the patient and explain the findings of the scan and ask for consent. I would inform the anaesthetist and the theatre coordinator and speak to the ITU registrar as the patient would need an HDU bed in the post-operative setting.

- Probes
  - What is the diagnosis?
  - Can she be managed conservatively?
  - Does she need a CT for the abdomen and pelvis

- Positive markers
  - Uses A–E assessment along with the assessment of operation notes and chart review
  - Understands the importance of excluding underlying causes of delirium, such as sepsis from an anastomotic leak.
  - Appropriately escalates
- Negative markers
  - Gives the patient sedatives without excluding causes for delirium
  - Does not work up the patient appropriately
  - Does not escalate

Urology

Clinical Scenario 16: Haematuria

You are the core surgical trainee in urology. A 65-year-old woman presents with a three-week history of painless, frank haematuria. Her medical history is significant for hypertension. She has a 40-pack-year history of smoking. How would you approach this patient?

I am concerned that this patient might have cancer of the urinary tract, given her history of significant smoking and persistent painless haematuria. Pertaining to this, I am also mindful that the patient could develop clot retention from significant haematuria. I would make sure to rule out benign conditions, such as UTIs and renal stones as a cause of haematuria. The patient might or might not require admission to the hospital, based on my assessment.

I would approach the patient using a CCrISP approach and do an A–E assessment. If she is hemodynamically stable, then I would proceed by taking a detailed history. I would start by exploring the history of haematuria in detail, asking about volume, colour, and clots. I would ask about any associated urinary symptoms, such as dysuria, frequent urination, or pneumaturia. I would ask about pain. I would ask about any recent weight loss or night sweats to assess for B-symptoms related to cancers. I would ask about any history of UTIs, renal stones, or any other urinary problems. On examination, I am particularly looking for any obvious abnormal masses in the suprapubic region and the renal angle. I would examine the patient using a chaperone.

In terms of investigations, I would request for FBC, U&E, CRP, and clotting profile to assess the patient for anaemia, any signs of infection, and any indication of renal dysfunction. I would also send a cross-match to ensure that blood could be given if required.

In terms of microbiological investigations, I would review the urine dip to rule out any infection. If it is nitrite or leucocyte positive, I would ask for it to be sent for MC&S. At this stage, I am concerned that the patient has an underlying malignancy. I think she would need an urgent outpatient CT scan on a two-week wait pathway. She would also require a flexible cystoscopy with biopsy. If she has a significant clot burden and is at risk for clot retention, I would arrange for admission to the hospital, placement of a three-way catheter, and irrigation with normal saline. If I think her presentation is more suggestive of renal colic, I would arrange for a CT KUB.

Once I have assessed this patient, I would involve my registrar or consultant to determine whether she should be managed as an inpatient or outpatient. Although the diagnosis of malignancy is not yet confirmed, I would alert the outpatient urology nurses to keep an eye out for her investigations. She might need to be added to a multidisciplinary team meeting for discussion.

Throughout all of this, I understand that this might be a difficult and stressful situation for the patient and her family. I would keep the patient at the centre of care, communicating with her sensitively. Breaking bad news of a cancer diagnosis is a very sensitive conversation, and it is best to wait for confirmation of the diagnosis before making any statements such as this. I would discuss the timing of this conversation with my registrar and consultant.

- Probes
  - What is your differential diagnosis?
  - What are your priorities?
  - What other information would you gather?
  - Who else would you like to involve in this patient's care?
- Positive markers
  - Considers malignancy as the most likely diagnosis
  - Constructs a reasonable differential diagnosis
  - Requests appropriate investigations
  - Escalates to the registrar or consultant appropriately
  - Has a structured approach to patient assessment
- Negative markers
  - Has an unstructured approach to patient assessment
  - Does not involve the wider healthcare team
  - Breaks bad news without adequate information
  - Does not consider inpatient versus outpatient management

Clinical Scenario 17: Renal Colic

You are the core surgical trainee on urology. A 65-year-old gentleman pres-
ents to A&E with severe right-sided flank pain. His urine dip is positive for
blood +++. How will you approach this patient?

From the information at hand, the patient appears to be having renal colic.
I would attend to the patient early and make sure the patient is comfortable as renal colic is a very painful condition. I would liaise with my A&E
colleagues and make sure the patient is prescribed appropriate analgesia
and is comfortable while waiting to be seen. The patient could also have
obstructive uropathy causing sepsis. Although less likely, this could also
represent a ruptured AAA, which is a surgical emergency.

On arrival, I would ask the patient and make sure he is comfortable
and pain-free. If not, I would review the analgesia on the drug charts and
prescribe more if appropriate. If the patient is unwell, I would follow an
A–E approach using the CCrISP protocol. However, if the patient is stable,
I would proceed to take a detailed history and examination. I would then
ask about the pain, in particular asking about the onset, duration, and
character. I would enquire about any associated urinary problems and any
history of renal stones. Specifically, I would also ask about risk factors for
AAA, such as cardiovascular disease and any previous aortic ultrasounds.
Using a chaperone, I would perform a full abdominal examination, in particular looking for renal angle tenderness or a palpable AAA. I am also
looking to see if the patient is displaying signs of sepsis, such as tachycar-
dia or fever.

I would request relevant investigations, which would include FBC,
U&E, LFTs, CRP, and amylase. The urine dip has already been inspected
and shows +++ blood. If the patient is septic, I would also get blood cultures. Based on a diagnosis of presumed renal colic, I would organise a
CT KUB non-contrast in consultation with my registrar. If I am in any
doubt about the diagnosis, a CT of the abdomen/pelvis or a CT angiogram
might be other options.

If I am concerned that the patient is septic with obstructive pyelone-
phritis, I would initiate sepsis 6. This includes starting high-flow oxygen,
IV fluids, and IV antibiotics, and I would take blood cultures, check lactate, and monitor urine output.

The eventual management for this patient depends on his clinical
situation and the results of his CT scan. If he has a small renal stone and
well-controlled pain, he might be managed as an outpatient. If he has an
obstructing stone causing sepsis, he would require admission and decompression, either with a retrograde stent or nephrostomy. If the patient had
an alternative diagnosis, such as a ruptured AAA, this would require
emergency specialist management by the vascular surgery team.

Throughout this patient's assessment, I am cognizant of the team that I work within. If I had an FY1, I might delegate specific tasks to them, such as taking blood specimens or placing a catheter. I would escalate to my registrar or consultant based on clinical urgency. I would also involve nursing and speak to radiology for advice.

Throughout all this, I would keep the patient at the centre of care and make sure I communicate my thinking process and findings with him.

- Probes
  - What is your differential diagnosis?
  - What are your priorities?
  - What other information would you gather?
  - Who else would you like to involve in this patient's care?
- Positive markers
  - Considers renal colic as the most likely diagnosis
  - Constructs a reasonable differential diagnosis
  - Requests appropriate investigations
  - Escalates to the registrar or consultant appropriately
  - Has a structured approach to patient assessment
- Negative markers
  - Has an unstructured approach to patient assessment
  - Does not involve the wider healthcare team
  - Does not offer early analgesia
  - Does not escalate patient care

Clinical Scenario 18: Paraphimosis

You are the core surgical trainee on urology. You are asked to see a 56-year-old gentleman as a ward referral. He is POD#2 after a sigmoid colectomy. He still has a urinary catheter, which is draining clear urine. He complains of intense pain in his penis. How will you approach this patient?

Penile pain in a post-op patient with a properly functioning catheter would make me consider paraphimosis. Other possibilities include irritation from the catheter or urinary tract infection. This might require reduction, catheter removal/exchange, or antibiotics, depending on my patient assessment.

I would approach the patient using an A–E approach, using the CCrISP algorithm. In the absence of acute haemodynamic concerns, I would proceed to take a focused urological history and examination. I would ask about the nature of the pain, its onset, and any aggravating or relieving factors. I would ask for associated symptoms, such as dysuria or haematuria. I would examine his penis, with a chaperone present, to see if he has a paraphimosis or if there is blood at the urethral meatus. I would also examine the output of the catheter to see if the urine is cloudy or bloody.

I would review the patient's notes and blood work. In particular, I would look at the operative note to see why the catheter was placed, if the foreskin was replaced, and whether there are any reasons (such as injury to the bladder intra-operatively) that would mean the catheter should stay in place.

If I think the patient does indeed have paraphimosis, I would prescribe adequate analgesia. I know that paraphimosis could be reduced at the bedside by applying gentle pressure to the swollen foreskin along the penile shaft for a few minutes to reduce oedema and then replacing the foreskin in its place. Hypertonic solutions, such as 50% dextrose, could be applied topically to osmotically reduce oedema. This could also be performed using a penile block. At this point in my training, I do not feel comfortable performing this procedure independently, so I would alert my registrar so that we could perform this together. If this is not successful at the bedside, the patient might need to go to theatre for a reduction +/− dorsal slit under general anaesthesia. This would involve coordination with theatres and the anaesthetic team. If I think the patient has a urinary tract infection, I would consider catheter exchange/removal and antibiotics.

Finally, this is an event in which the patient has come to harm. I would submit a Datix form and discuss this case at morbidity and mortality for the whole team to learn lessons from this adverse event. I would also discuss this with the patient, using the duty of candour rules.

- Probes
  - What is your differential diagnosis?
  - What other information would you gather?
  - When would you escalate this patient's care?
  - If you find that the patient has paraphimosis, how would you proceed?
- Positive markers
  - Considers paraphimosis as the most likely diagnosis
  - Constructs a reasonable differential diagnosis
  - Escalates to the registrar or consultant appropriately
  - Has a structured approach to patient assessment
  - Understands own limitations
- Negative markers
  - Does not consider paraphimosis
  - Does not consider whether the urinary catheter needs to stay in place
  - Has an unstructured approach to patient assessment
  - Does not review analgesia
  - Does not escalate patient care

Clinical Scenario 19: Urinary Retention

You are the core surgical trainee on urology. A 57-year-old gentleman presents to A&E with the inability to pass urine for the past 12 hours. He is now in significant discomfort. He is otherwise fit and well. How will you approach this patient?

The patient appears to be in urinary retention. I would ask A&E to do a bladder scan to confirm this diagnosis. The patient might require a catheter and possible admission for monitoring of fluid fluxes. Another differential is hypovolaemia with resultant low urinary output, with the pain being caused by an alternative intra-abdominal pathology.

I would assess the patient using the CCrISP guidelines. Once I am satisfied with the A–E assessment and I have confirmed that the patient is hemodynamically stable, I would proceed to assess for acute urine retention. I would take a detailed history and specifically ask about any urinary tract symptoms, such as dysuria or frequent urination. I would try to establish if the patient has pre-existing prostatic symptoms, such as dribbling. On examination, I would feel for a distended, palpable, tender bladder and try to exclude any other cause for acute abdominal pain. With a chaperone present, I would also perform a digital rectal examination to assess the prostrate for enlargement.

In terms of investigations, I would get an FBC, CRP, U&E, LFTs, amylase, and PSA. This would enable me to assess renal function and other causes of abdominal pain. The bladder scan would show me if there indeed is retention. If the bladder scan shows >500 ml of urine, I would catheterise the patient. Concomitantly, I would send a urine dip and send urine for MCS.

I would escalate to my registrar if I am unable to catheterise the patient as I do not want to cause traumatic urethral injury through multiple attempts. The patient might require a supra-public catheter or a flexible cystoscopy-assisted catheter insertion over a guide wire. I could not perform these procedures currently but would be interested to learn from my seniors. I would also discuss with my senior if an ultrasound KUB would be of value for this patient. Depending on the patient's clinical status, we might be able to manage this in an outpatient setting, in which case I would liaise with the urology clinic to arrange for follow-up in the TWOC clinic. Alternatively, I might need to liaise with nursing and bed management to get a bed for this patient if the patient is being admitted as an inpatient.

I would keep the patient at the centre of care, especially as having a catheter might be uncomfortable for him.

- Probes
  - What is your diagnosis?
  - What other information would you gather?

- How would you escalate this patient's care?
- If you fail to catheterise the patient, what other options would you consider?
- Positive markers
  - Considers urinary retention as the most likely diagnosis
  - Constructs a reasonable differential diagnosis
  - Escalates to the registrar or consultant appropriately
  - Has a structured approach to patient assessment
  - Understands own limitations
- Negative markers
  - Does not attend to the patient and delegates management to A&E
  - Has an unstructured approach to patient assessment
  - Does not escalate patient care
  - Is not aware of other options if urethral catheterisation fails

Clinical Scenario 20: Testicular Torsion

You are the core surgical trainee on urology. A 12-year-old boy presents with a four-hour history of sudden, severe left testicular pain. The pain started while he was playing volleyball. How will you approach this patient?

Given the age and presentation, I am concerned about testicular torsion, which is a surgical emergency. The other differential is testicular trauma. As such, my priority would be to quickly assess the patient, and if I am suspecting testicular torsion, then I would urgently escalate to my registrar since the patient needs to go to theatre for scrotal exploration within six hours of the onset of pain.

I would assess this patient immediately using the CCrISP algorithm. If he has haemodynamically stable, I would take a focused history and examination. I would specifically ask about the onset of pain and timing. I would ask about any associated trauma or swelling. I would ask about pre-existing lumps or bumps. On examination, I would use a chaperone and ask for permission for a genital examination. Specifically, I would look for a tender, high-riding testicle with the absence of a cremasteric reflex.

Testicular torsion is a clinical diagnosis and requires no further investigations. A urine dip might be helpful to exclude a UTI or epididymo-orchitis. If I found a scrotal haematoma on the background of trauma, I might request an ultrasound of the scrotum. I would make this decision in close collaboration with my registrar or consultant, whom I would involve early in this case.

If the patient needs to go to theatre, then I would communicate this with the theatre staff, on-call anaesthetist, and A&E. This might also require communication with other surgical specialities who share CEPOD theatres as the case order might need to change. Sometimes a second theatre might need to be opened up. If I feel competent, I would consent the patient for scrotal exploration and mark the correct side with a permanent marker.

I am conscious that this is a stressful, high-stakes situation. The patient and his family might be concerned about the viability of the testicle, and I would do my utmost to keep them at the centre of our care and informed every step of the way.

- Probes
  - What are your priorities?
  - What other information would you gather?
  - How would you escalate this patient's care?
  - If the patient required an emergency scrotal exploration, whom would you need to inform?
- Positive markers
  - Appreciates the urgency of the situation and attends to the patient immediately
  - Recognises that this requires a team-based approach
  - Escalates to the registrar or consultant appropriately
  - Books patient for theatre and discusses with theatre team and anaesthesia
- Negative markers
  - Does not attend immediately
  - Uses an unstructured approach to patient assessment
  - Does not escalate patient care
  - Fails to book the patient for theatre properly
  - Does not recognise testicular torsion or its urgency

ENT

Clinical Scenario 21: Neck Mass

> *You are the ENT SHO asked to review a 40-year-old lady who has presented to A&E with a neck mass. She complains of a two-month history of 'tightness' in her neck. She denies pain or breathlessness but feels that over the previous fortnight, she can feel a more palpable mass on the front of her neck.*

Neck masses encompass a broad range of differentials, both benign and malignant. I am concerned that this patient might have a thyroid, parathyroid, or lymphatic malignancy. Benign diagnoses could include thyroid or parathyroid masses, infection, Graves' disease, Hashimoto's thyroiditis, and lymphadenopathy secondary to an infection. With a rapid increase in size, I would attend to the patient urgently, particularly to ensure her airway is secure.

I would assess the patient using the CCrISP algorithm. If she was hae-modynamically stable, I would undertake a thorough and detailed history with focused questions about thyroid/parathyroid imbalance, such as weight loss or gain, heat or cold intolerance, diarrhoea or constipation, excessive sweating, tremors, lethargy, palpitations, visual disturbance, and menstrual irregularities. I would specifically ask about any red flag symptoms, including unintentional weight loss, loss of appetite, night sweats, difficult or painful swallowing, and voice change/hoarseness. I would ask about any fever, localised pain, and any swallowing difficulties. I would then inquire about the patient's smoking status, use of alcohol and any other illicit drugs, and radiation exposure and also gather information about her family history with a focus on any autoimmune, thyroid/parathyroid, and endocrine pathologies.

I would then get a full set of observations and review them, with emphasis on pulse rate, blood pressure, and temperature. I would then carefully examine the patient. This would include a quick general physical exam followed by a thorough examination of the neck swelling from behind. The examination would involve careful inspection to ascertain the position, size, symmetry, extent, and shape of the swelling followed by palpation to ascertain firmness, regularity, mobility, and tenderness, as well as tracheal position. I would then ask the patient to stick her tongue out, followed by swallowing, and look for any associated movement of the swelling, I would also auscultate the mass for any bruits and check for any neck vein distention. I would finish the examination by looking for common signs associated with thyroid pathology, such as exophthalmos, lid lag, tremors, pretibial myxoedema, and loss of lateral eyebrows. I would keep a broad differential while assessing the patient in case my differential changes, such as a vascular lesion or muscular mass.

This patient needs blood tests, including FBC, U&E, LFTs, bone profile, thyroid functions tests (including T3, free T4, and TSH), and parathyroid hormone levels. With the blood tests available, I would discuss this patient with my on-call registrar.

If the patient has a thyroid emergency, such as thyroid storm, I would start oxygen, IV fluids, and paracetamol. I would liaise with the medical registrar on-call regarding starting beta blockers and anti-thyroid medications. This patient might require a higher level of care, in which case I would liaise with the HDU team.

Alternatively, if the patient is not acutely unwell and does not require hospital admission, I would arrange for an urgent two-week-wait ultrasound of her neck +/− FNA. I would alert the outpatient ENT team to keep an eye on this result and make arrangements for the patient's results to be reviewed in a timely manner.

I would explain the management plan to the patient and answer any questions she might have.

- Probes
  - What are your immediate concerns?
  - What are your differentials?
  - What other information would you gather?
  - How would you escalate this patient's care?
- Positive markers
  - Takes thorough and focused history
  - Considers benign and malignant causes for presentation
  - Considers conditions requiring hospital admission
  - Requests relevant investigations (TFTs, bone profile)
  - Recognises the need for USS and FNAC
- Negative markers
  - Uses an unstructured approach
  - Fails to rule out emergency conditions
  - Does not take a focused history
  - Is not mindful of malignancy
  - Does not request appropriate blood tests
  - Fails to involve senior

Clinical Scenario 22: Bleeding Post-Thyroidectomy

You are the core surgical trainee on-call at a tertiary teaching hospital. You are asked to see a 41-year-old lady in theatre recovery for dyspnoea. She is freshly post-hemithyroidectomy for a thyroid nodule. Her left neck is grossly swollen. How would you approach this patient?

I am most concerned this patient might be suffering from a post-operative haematoma, causing airway obstruction, though unilateral laryngeal nerve injury is also a differential. I would advise the recovery staff to apply high-flow oxygen and obtain a full set of observations. I would attend to the patient immediately, and if the operating surgeon were still present, I would inform them as well.

I would evaluate the patient using a CCrISP approach. On immediate assessment, I would assess for patency of the airway by speaking to the patient. I would listen for the patient's upper airway sounds, listening for stridor, hoarseness, or 'breathy' sounds. I would also inspect the neck, assessing for any swelling, bruising, leaking staple lines, and tracheal deviation. Were there any of these findings, I would inform my senior immediately as this is a surgical emergency. In extremis and in the absence of immediate available help, I would take a systematic approach to open the wound at the bedside, by exposing skin, cutting sutures, opening the skin, opening superficial and deep layers of muscle, evacuating the haematoma, and packing the wound. This would relieve pressure on the trachea causing airway obstruction. I would then re-evaluate the airway and proceed to do the A–E assessment. If the clinical acuity of the patient allows, I would also read the operative note to determine if there has been any concern over haemostasis.

After the procedure, the patient would need an immediate return to theatre for haemostasis, so early contact with the on-call anaesthetist, specifically informing them of airway compromise and potentially distorted anatomy, would allow them to prepare their theatre and airway equipment to allow safe intubation. The operating surgeon or the on-call ENT/general/endocrine surgeon (depending on the provision of these specialities at the local site) would need to be informed of their assistance in the operation. Post-operatively, the patient might require a high-dependency unit or intensive care unit bed, so liaison with the critical care team would aid post-operative destination planning.

Given this was an unplanned return to theatre, there has to be a duty of candour discussion with the patient post-operatively. The patient also needs to be discussed in the departmental morbidity and mortality meeting.

- Probes
  - What are your priorities?
  - What are your differentials for post-surgical dyspnoea?
  - When will you involve your seniors?
- Positive markers
  - Attends to the patient immediately
  - Recognises this is a life-threatening emergency
  - Suggests opening of the surgical wound to evacuate the haematoma
  - Considers forward destination beyond initial management
- Negative markers
  - Does not attend immediately
  - Has an unstructured approach
  - Does not escalate
  - Fails to consider definitive management

Clinical Scenario 23: Epistaxis

You are the core-surgical trainee and are called to see a 50-year-old man with a background of hypertension and atrial fibrillation on ramipril and warfarin. He presents to ED with active epistaxis from the left nostril. How would you proceed?

The most common causes of epistaxis include trauma, hypertension, or secondary to drugs such as anticoagulants or antiplatelets. I would enquire about when the bleeding started, and how much blood he has lost. I would also ask if there was any history of recurrent epistaxis, bruising, or bleeding from elsewhere.

I would immediately go and see the patient and assess him using the ABCDE approach. I would assess the airway by speaking to the patient. If they were speaking in clear full sentences, I would give 15 litre of oxygen via a non-rebreathe mask and move onto breathing.

The priority in this patient is to arrest the bleeding and ensure he is haemodynamically stable. I would assess his pulse, cap refill, and blood pressure. I would ask for help with IV access with a large bore cannula and simultaneously take blood including VBG, FBC, U&E, LFT, CRP, group and screen, and clotting.

I would then start fluid resuscitation and ask for help from one of the nursing staff to apply pressure to the soft part of the nose of the patient for 15 minutes while they were sitting forward. If this does not arrest the bleed, I would then proceed to pack the nose with either an absorbable pack or a rapid rhino which could apply haemostatic pressure.

I would consider warfarin reversal if the bleeding restarts and discuss this patient with haematology.

I would escalate this patient to the registrar on call, as the patient may need to be taken to theatre for cauterisation of the bleed, if the bleeding does not stop with packing.

Once the bleeding has stopped, the nasal pack would stay in situ for at least 24 hours prior to removal and consideration of discharge.

I would ensure I speak to the patient and their family to ensure they are informed of the management and answer any questions they may have.

- Probes
    - What further information do you need?
    - What tests do you require?
    - Will you reverse the warfarin?
- Positive markers
    - Assess using ABCDE approach
    - Needs IV access as a matter of urgency
    - Requests appropriate initial investigations including G&S and FBC
    - If ongoing bleeding should be escalated and prepared for theatre
- Negative markers
    - Does not prioritise this patient
    - Unstructured approach
    - Does not escalate patient

Clinical Scenario 24: Peritonsillar Abscess

You are a core surgical trainee and are called to see a 30-year-old women with a history of tonsillitis presented to the emergency department. On this occasion, she cannot speak properly and has been unable to swallow any tablets or eat food due to the pain. You are asked to come and assess the patient to rule out a peritonsillar abscess.

In this scenario, I am concerned this patient has a peritonsillar abscess. I would assess her using an ABCDE approach. First, I would speak to the patient to assess her airway status. If she cannot speak to me in full sentences, I will conduct a airway assessment before moving on. I would do this by examining the oral cavity, to assess the tonsils for any obvious peritonsillar swelling or deviation of the uvula. If this is present, then the most important treatment to secure the airway is aspiration of the abscess to remove pus and create more space. I will consider escalating to the anaesthetic team early if my patient needs airway support.

I would then move on to assess breathing and circulation. I would assess the pulse rate and blood pressure and secure IV access for further treatment. I would take blood including VBG, FBC, U&E, LFT, CRP, and clotting. I would start fluid resuscitation, intravenous antibiotics, and give a stat dose of steroid to help reduce swelling.

I would ensure that the patient has a full range of neck movements as it is important to ensure there are no signs of a deep neck space infection. I will also check the patient's GCS.

After completing my examination, I would admit the patient for IV fluids, regular IV antibiotics, and steroids. I would escalate the patient to the registrar on call in case further aspiration or incision and drainage of the abscess is required.

I would speak to the patient and their family to ensure they are informed of the management and answer any questions they may have.

Once the patient can eat and drink and swallow tablets they can be discharged to complete a course of oral antibiotics.

- Probes
  - What is the priority for this patient?
  - What is the most important treatment?
- Positive markers
  - Assess using ABCDE approach
  - Airway is assessed appropriately
  - Peritonsillar abscess is aspirated
- Negative markers
  - Does not rule out deep neck space infection
  - Does not start on IV antibiotics
  - Does not escalate patient

Plastics

Clinical Scenario 25: Necrotising Fasciitis

You are the SHO on-call for plastics and have been asked to see a 35-year-old female IVDU who presents three days after injecting heroin into her right wrist. She has severe pain around the injection site. The pain has been getting worse with increased erythema, redness, and tracking up the arm. She is febrile, tachycardic, and hypotensive. How would you approach this patient?

I am the SHO on-call for plastics and have been asked to see a 35-year-old intravenous drug user who is presenting with pain in her wrist. She is potentially showing signs of septic shock. Given how sick she is, I would inform my registrar of the referral. Over the phone, I would ask the ED to initiate the sepsis 6 protocol. My current differentials are necrotising fasciitis, complicated cellulitis, abscess, or a foreign body like a needle in the forearm. She might require theatre.

I would approach the patient using the CCrISP protocol. If the patient could speak to me, her airways are patent. I would then want to know her respiratory rate and oxygen saturation and ensure she was on high-flow oxygen if clinically indicated. I would assess breathing by inspecting if the patient is in respiratory distress. I would feel for any signs of tracheal deviation and unequal chest expansion and percuss the lungs bilaterally. I would then auscultate the lungs anteriorly and posteriorly to assess for equal air entry. If the airway is intact, I would move on to circulation. I would assess the patient's heart rate, blood pressure, and fluid status. I would ensure that the patient has two large-bore cannulas inserted where I would take an FBC, U&E, CRP, LFTS, coagulation screen, and group and save. I would take an ABG to assess the patient's lactate level. In addition, I would commence the sepsis 6 protocol by taking blood cultures, monitoring the urine output, administering fluids and antibiotics, taking the patient's lactate level, and giving oxygen if needed. Finally, in circulation, I would ensure an ECG is done as the patient is tachycardic. If circulation is now stable, I would move on to disability by assessing the patient's GCS, blood glucose levels from my ABG, and temperature. Lastly, I would expose the patient appropriately, assessing her from head to toe but focusing on the right arm.

On the right arm, I would inspect for signs of erythema, abscesses, open wounds, and track marks. At this point, I would mark out the patient's erythema. I would feel for any signs of crepitus, warmth, and tenderness and assess how soft or firm the compartments are. As I am most concerned about necrotising fasciitis, I would perform the sweep test and look for signs of discoloured water. This completes my A–E assessment. At this point, I would ensure that my registrar is aware of the situation and take a focused history. I might also consider an x-ray of the forearm if I am concerned about a retained foreign object, such as a needle.

If the patient has necrotising fasciitis, then she requires definitive management with operative debridement. As the SHO, I would prepare the patient for theatre by ensuring that the patient is nil by mouth and has been booked onto the CEPOD list and that the on-call anaesthetist is aware. I would ensure that antibiotics are started after discussion with microbiology. The first-line treatment for necrotising fasciitis in my unit is benzylpenicillin with clindamycin. Furthermore, I would inform the ITU/HDU about this patient as she might go there post-operatively for inotropic or vasopressor support.

I appreciate that this must be a stressful situation for the patient, and I would update her and her next of kin about the urgency and severity of the situation.

- Probes
  - What is your differential diagnosis?
  - How would you escalate this patient's care?
  - What features in this presentation make you think about sepsis?
  - What definitive care would you offer this patient?
- Positive markers
  - Appreciates the urgency of the situation and attends to the patient immediately
  - Considers life-threatening diagnoses, such as necrotising fasciitis
  - Recognises that seniors should be involved early
  - Assesses the patient with a structured approach
- Negative markers
  - Does not consider the life-threatening condition early on
  - Uses an unstructured approach
  - Escalates at the end of the scenario rather than early
  - Does not recognise septic shock

Clinical Scenario 26: Burns

You are the SHO on plastics. You have been asked to see a 26-year-old male who presents to A&E via ambulance with partial-thickness burns to his face, trunk, and left arm following a house fire in an enclosed space. How would you approach this patient?

I am concerned that this patient has had extensive burns following a house fire. The burns to the face could lead to inhalation injuries and a compromised airway. The trunk burns, if circumferential, could contribute to respiratory distress. In any trauma call, I would also be concerned about other traumatic injuries. I would attend to this patient immediately.

I would put out a trauma call immediately. I would inform my registrar of this situation.

I would approach the patient using an ATLS approach. I would ensure that his c-spine is secured with three-point immobilisation. I would assess her airway by first speaking to him and starting high-flow oxygen. At the same time, I would look for any signs of soot inhalation around the nostrils and mouth, as well as any signs of stridor. If the patient has signs of airway compromise, this could require intubation, and I would alert the anaesthetic team immediately.

At breathing, I would want to know the patient's respiratory rate and oxygen saturation. I would look for signs of respiratory distress, paying particular attention to the patient's chest to check for circumferential burns. If this is the case, the patient might need an escharotomy. Next, I would feel if the trachea is central, check for equal chest expansion anteriorly and posteriorly, and percuss the lungs. I would then auscultate to hear for equal breath sounds bilaterally. I would ask my FY1 to obtain an ABG and also use this sample to obtain carboxyhaemoglobin levels.

If the airway is intact, I would move on to circulation, with my main concern here being fluid resuscitation and any signs of haemorrhage from the five main areas from concomitant trauma. I would want to know the patient's heart rate and blood pressure. I would assess the patient's fluid status and insert two large-bore cannulas. I would send for a full blood count, U&E, LFTs, CK, and cross-match. I would start 1 litre of Hartman's stat and insert a urinary catheter to monitor fluid output. If circulation is stable, I would move on to disability by assessing the patient's GCS, blood glucose, and temperature.

Lastly, I would expose the patient from head to toe, looking for any additional injuries. I would ask the nursing staff to completely remove the patient's clothing to stop the burning process whilst preventing overexposure and hypothermia.

This completes my primary survey. My secondary survey would involve calculating the total body surface area (TBSA) burnt using Wallace's rule of nines and calculating how much fluids to give over a 24-hour period using the Parkland formula.

My immediate investigations would have been done in the primary survey. At this point, I would want to inform my registrar who would be part of the trauma call and my consultant. If the main issues only relate to burns, this patient should be transferred to a specialised burn unit, and I would facilitate this. I might need to involve anaesthetics for airway control, general surgery if I find any other life-threatening injuries, and orthopaedics for orthopaedic injuries. Depending on my assessment, the patient might also require further investigations, such as a trauma CT scan.

During all of this, I would keep the patient at the centre of care. I would ensure that he is receiving adequate analgesia as burns could be very painful. If possible, I would also explore the circumstances around the burn and consider whether this is an accident, self-harm attempt, or assault.

- Probes
  - In a burn patient who has had both facial and trunk burns, what additional pathologies are you most worried about?
  - How would you escalate this patient's care?
  - Who else would you involve in this patient's care?
- Positive markers
  - Appreciates the urgency of the situation and attends to the patient immediately
  - Puts out a trauma call immediately and involves the plastics team
  - Recognises that seniors should be involved early
  - Assesses the patient using a structured ATLS approach
  - Is aware of when to fluid-resuscitate a patient
  - Mentions Parkland formula for fluid resuscitation
  - Mentions Wallace's rule of nines to estimate burn severity
- Negative markers
  - Does not attend immediately
  - Uses an unstructured approach to patient assessment
  - Fails to include other members of the trauma team
  - Does not escalate patient care
  - Does not recognise the patient might have suffered inhalation injuries or circumferential burns
  - Does not initiate fluid resuscitation

Clinical Scenario 27: Dog Bite

You are the SHO on-call for plastics, and you are asked to see a 53-year-old female dogwalker who got bit on the palmar surface of her right index finger this morning. She comes into the ED complaining of swelling and stiffness of the right index finger. How would you approach this patient?

I am concerned that this patient has had a dog bite, which could lead to an infection, such as a deep space infection or a flexor sheath infection. I am also concerned about the potential for neurovascular and bone injuries.

I would assess the patient following the CCrISP protocol. If the patient is speaking to me, her airway is patent, and I am happy to move on to breathing. In breathing, I want to know the patient's respiratory rate and oxygen saturation and if clinically indicated I would start her on 15 litres of oxygen with a non-rebreather mask. I would assess her breathing by looking to see if she is in respiratory distress. I would then feel her trachea and check for equal chest expansion bilaterally followed by auscultation. If breathing is stable, I would move on to circulation. Here, I would want to know the patient's heart rate, blood pressure, and temperature. I would assess her fluid status and insert a large-bore cannula. I would take an FBC, U&E, CRP, LFTs, coagulation screen, VBG, and group and save. If the patient shows any signs of sepsis, I would instigate the septic 6 protocol of taking blood cultures, monitoring the urinary output, administering fluids, starting broad-spectrum antibiotics, measuring the lactate level, and starting oxygen. If circulation is stable, I would assess the patient's disability by checking her GCS, blood sugar levels, and temperature. I would expose the patient, focusing my examination on her hand.

On examination, I would be looking for any signs of puncture wounds, swelling, erythema, pus, discharge, and if the finger is in a fixed flexed position. I would then feel if the hand is hot and assess areas of tenderness, especially along the flexor sheath. This would be followed by a neurovascular examination, which would involve assessing the hand's function.

Following my CCrISP assessment, I would take a focused history regarding hand dominance, time of onset, and any medical history leading to poor wound healing, such as the presence of diabetes or taking steroids. An x-ray of the hand in two views would be needed to ensure there are no underlying fractures. Once I have all this information, I would escalate to my registrar about my findings.

To manage this patient effectively, she would need to be admitted into the hospital for intravenous antibiotics and formal washout and debridement in theatre. As the SHO, I would facilitate this process by informing the on-call anaesthetist, booking on the CEPOD list, and ensuring all the relevant blood specimens have been sent. If I feel confident, I would get consent from the patient and mark her. I would also inform the on-call consultant.

I appreciate that this might be a stressful situation for the patient, and I would keep her informed every step of the way.

- Probes
  - What are your differentials?
  - Which structures are you most concerned about being damaged?
  - What further investigations would you request?
- Positive markers
  - Appreciates the urgency of the situation and attends to the patient immediately
  - Escalates appropriately
  - Assesses the patient with a structured approach

- Negative markers
  - Does not admit the patient
  - Uses an unstructured approach
  - Fails to escalate care
  - Does not coordinate emergency washout

Orthopaedics

Clinical Scenario 28: Hip Fracture

You are the core surgical trainee on-call for orthopaedics. You have been asked by A&E to see a 92-year-old lady who had a fall at home. She was on the floor for five hours before being found. She is in A&E with an externally rotated leg.

In this scenario, I am concerned about a fractured neck of femur. She might also have acute kidney injury secondary to rhabdomyolysis, given her prolonged lying on the floor. Additionally, I am also concerned about hypothermia, given this patient's age and prolonged lying. She might require operative intervention for her hip fracture.

This is a trauma patient who should be treated using an ATLS approach. However, given the nature of the referral, it is possible that A&E might already have performed a primary survey and possibly cleared the c-spine. If this was the case, then I would proceed to review the patient's observations and available investigations, as well as the A&E clerking. I would also make note of the patient's comorbidities and drug history.

I would take a full history from the patient herself, finding out the mechanism of the fall – was it mechanical or non-mechanical? I would want to know of any preceding symptoms, such as chest pain, shortness of breath, or neurological symptoms that might explain the cause of her fall. I would ask about the location of her pain and discomfort.

I would then examine the patient. I would speak to her, and receiving a response would ensure her airway is patent and self-maintained. I would then look at her breathing and feel for any asymmetrical chest movement or crepitus in the chest wall, auscultating the chest for any abnormal breath sounds, measuring the respiratory rate and oxygen saturation levels. If she is hypoxic or tachypnoeic, then I would start oxygen supplementation.

I would move to assess the patient's circulation, looking for any signs of hypotension or impaired perfusion. I would feel for her central and peripheral pulses for rate, rhythm, character, and volume. I would auscultate the precordium for abnormal heart sounds and then measure her heart rate, blood pressure, capillary refill time, and temperature. I would request an ECG to exclude an arrhythmia as the cause of her fall.

I would cannulate her, to take baseline blood tests such as FBC, U&E, LFTs, clotting, and two group and save samples. This is because this patient is highly likely to require an operation for her neck of femur fracture, so knowing her clotting function is within normal limits is important, and she might require a transfusion (either pre-operatively to optimise or post-operatively due to blood loss). She should also have no food for six hours and no clear fluids for two hours pre-operatively so the cannula would allow administration of medications during her nil-by-mouth period. She should also have a CK to assess for rhabdomyolysis.

I would then assess the patient's consciousness using the Glasgow coma scale and also request a blood glucose measurement.

I would fully expose the patient and examine her fully, including a dedicated musculoskeletal examination of the affected hip and any other joints that might have been injured. I would also assess the neurovascular status of any affected limbs.

After the full examination, I would determine if any further investigations are required in addition to the blood tests requested. If no imaging has been completed, then a plain x-ray of the pelvis, affected hip, and femur would be required, as well as any other injured limbs. If urine or chest infection could be considered the cause of the patient's fall, then a urine dip and chest x-ray would be indicated.

If the fractured neck of femur is confirmed, then the patient would benefit from a fascia iliaca block for pain relief before definitive fixation of her fracture.

Given the prolonged lying, I am concerned about an acute kidney injury. This could be secondary to rhabdomyolysis. The treatment for this is usually intravenous fluids.

Once I have made an assessment, I would involve my registrar or consultant. I think the patient would require definitive treatment of her fracture, and this would need to be coordinated. I would escalate across to other specialities, such as the renal registrar and medical registrar, to get advice for the AKI and potentially to treat any cardiac or neurological causes for the patient's fall. I would inform the ITU registrar after discussion with the renal/medical team in case the patient needs haemofiltration prior to surgery. I would also inform the anaesthetic registrar and the theatre coordinator as this patient would need surgical fixation. Finally, I would involve the orthogeriatric team as this patient would need their input.

I would then document my findings and management plan and complete a drug chart including the patient's regular medications, analgesia, VTE prophylaxis, and intravenous fluids. If the registrar is happy for me to ask consent from the patient, then I would discuss the operation with the patient, complete the consent form, mark the affected side, and book her on the next available trauma list.

I understand that this is a stressful situation for the patient. I would call the patient's family and inform them of the plan. Given the patient's advanced age, if she has carers, they need to be informed. Given that the patient lay for a long time before being found, it is also possible that the patient has safeguarding issues and might not be able to manage at home any longer going forward.

- Probes
  - What is your differential diagnosis?
  - What are your priorities?
  - What other information would you gather?
  - Who else would you like to involve in this patient's care?
- Positive markers
  - Recognises the risk of AKI and rhabdomyolysis
  - Manages analgesia appropriately
  - Involves appropriate specialities
- Negative markers
  - Requests A&E to do the x-ray and re-refer if fractured
  - Fails to understand the importance of managing the AKI prior to surgery

Clinical Scenario 29: Cauda Equina Syndrome

You are the core surgical trainee on orthopaedics. You are asked to review a 32-year-old male manual worker in A&E. He complains of a two-day history of lumbar back pain and bilateral leg pain. Since this morning, he has had difficulty passing urine and an altered sensation in his perineum. How would you manage this patient?

I am concerned that this patient has a spinal emergency like cauda equina syndrome. He has back and leg pain with difficulty passing urine and altered sensation in his perineum. I would review this patient urgently. He would likely require an urgent MRI and possibly spinal decompression.

I would examine this patient using a CCrISP approach, doing an initial A–E assessment and reading the A&E notes. Then I would obtain a detailed history of the back/leg pain and inquire about any incontinence and altered perianal sensation. I would ask about recent trauma. I would enquire about medical history, medications, and allergies.

After providing adequate analgesia, I would perform a complete neurological examination of the lower limbs. This exam would include straight leg raise to test sciatic stretch. I would test for tone, sensation, and power in the lower limbs. For sensation, I would assess light touch and pin prick. I would assess the patient's lower-limb reflexes, including knee jerk, ankle jerk, and Babinski. I would perform a PR exam with a chaperone. I would test for tone and sensation – again light and pinprick. I would ask for a pre-void and post-void bladder scan.

I would gain IV access and obtain initial blood tests (FBC, U&E, CRP, and ESR). Since I am concerned about cauda equina, I would ask radiology for an urgent MRI scan.

I would inform my registrar of my findings. Pending the results of the MRI, I might also need to involve anaesthetics and the theatre team.

I would explain the potential diagnosis and management plan to the patient. Cauda equina syndrome is the compression of the cauda equina nerve roots that leads to the development of back or leg pain, lower-limb neurological deficit, saddle anaesthesia, and bladder or bowel dysfunction. The urinary incontinence is from overflow due to retention. The patient should be kept nil by mouth until a final read is available on the MRI. Surgical intervention in the form of emergency spinal decompression would be required.

- Probes
  - What are your concerns with this patient?
  - How would examine this patient?
  - How would you further investigate this patient?
  - How would you escalate this patient's care?
- Positive markers
  - Appreciates the urgency of the situation
  - Performs a neurological examination, including PR
  - Organises an urgent MRI scan
  - Asks for a pre- and post-void bladder scan
  - Escalates appropriately
- Negative markers
  - Does not attend to the patient urgently
  - Has an unstructured approach to examination
  - Uses inappropriate or inadequate investigations
  - Does not escalate urgently

Clinical Scenario 30: Shoulder Dislocation

You are the core surgical trainee for orthopaedics. You attend to an 18-year-old rugby player in A&E who was tackled and fell onto his right shoulder. He experienced immediate pain and is unable to move his shoulder despite analgesia. How would you approach this patient?

Considering the mechanism of injury and the patient's inability to move his shoulder, I suspect a shoulder dislocation. A dislocated joint is an orthopaedic emergency and needs early, safe reduction.

I would approach this patient using an ATLS approach. Given the nature of this referral, I would presume that A&E has already done a primary survey and perhaps cleared the c-spine. However, I would still perform a quick A–E assessment to exclude any other concomitant life-threatening injuries. If the patient is haemodynamically stable with an isolated complaint, then I would focus on the shoulder.

I would first provide this patient with adequate analgesia and then obtain a brief history of the mechanism of injury and any previous fractures or dislocations to this shoulder. My examination would include noting the position of the arm – abducted and externally rotated if anterior dislocation and internally rotated if posterior dislocation. I would perform a neurovascular assessment of the affected limb and compare it to the contralateral side. I found focus my neurological examination on the affected limb, looking at tone, power, sensation, and reflexes. The examination would be limited in some aspects by the inability to move the shoulder. I would assess the vascular status by feeling for distal pulses and measuring capillary refill time.

An urgent x-ray is required for confirmation of the diagnosis and to also ascertain if a concurrent fracture has been sustained. The x-rays should include two orthogonal views. Dislocations could be anterior or posterior. Anterior dislocations constitute the majority of shoulder dislocations. Posterior dislocations could often be initially missed. When reviewing x-rays, I would look for the 'light bulb' sign, which indicates posterior dislocation.

At this stage, I would escalate this patient's care to my registrar. If a simple dislocation is found, then closed reduction in A&E using adequate analgesia should be attempted. Multiple attempts at reduction should be avoided as this could lead to fractures and neurovascular injuries. The manoeuvre for reduction is the traction-countertraction method.

Once the joint is reduced, neurovascular assessment and x-ray must be repeated. A referral to the physiotherapy team is important.

In the case of an irreducible dislocation or if there is a concomitant fracture, this patient would require urgent manipulation under anaesthesia in theatre. Hence, the patient should be nil by mouth. I would prepare the consent form for my registrar and mark the appropriate side. I would also involve my consultant, the anaesthetist, and theatre team. The patient should be aware of the risk of requiring and open surgical reduction for dislocations that fail closed procedure.

Throughout this process, I would keep the patient at the centre of care. I would communicate our decision-making to him and make sure he is involved in all decision-making. I realise that performing a closed reduction in A&E could be traumatic for the patient, and I would do my utmost to make sure he is reassured and receives adequate analgesia or sedation.

- Probes
  - What are your concerns with this patient?
  - How would you examine this patient?
  - How would you investigate this patient?

- Positive markers
  - Provides adequate analgesia
  - Performs a neurovascular examination
  - Obtains basic imaging (x-ray)
  - Escalates patient care to the registrar appropriately
- Negative markers
  - Does not appreciate the variety and complexity of potential injuries
  - Does not provide adequate analgesia
  - Proceeds with manipulation without initial imaging
  - Does not escalate patient care

Clinical Scenario 31: Compartment Syndrome

You are the core surgical trainee for orthopaedics. A 27-year-old male cyclist sustained a closed right tibial fracture. He has been admitted for overnight analgesia and tibial intramedullary nailing the following morning. He is tachycardic and in severe pain in his right leg. How would you approach this patient?

I am concerned that this patient has compartment syndrome following tibial fracture. This is an orthopaedic emergency, and I would attend this patient immediately.

I would review the patient using a CCrISP approach. I would perform a quick A–E assessment of the patient. If there are no life-threatening issues, I would proceed to focus on the affected limb.

I would review the observation chart, paying attention to the pain score and review the drug chart for analgesia taken so far. If inadequate analgesia has been administered, then I would proceed to prescribe some urgently. Otherwise, I would take down any bandages or split any back slab that has been applied and elevate the limb. I would proceed to examine the affected limb. I would do a full neurovascular and musculoskeletal examination. In particular, I am looking for pain out of proportion on passive stretch. This would indicate compartment syndrome, which is a clinical diagnosis. From a neurological point of view, altered sensation or paraesthesia could indicate nerve damage. From a vascular point of view, lack of a peripheral pulse and paralysis are late findings and carry a very poor prognosis. I do not think that any further investigations are warranted at this point.

I would immediately escalate to the orthopaedic registrar or consultant. I would also make the patient nil by mouth, gain adequate IV access, take initial blood specimens (FBC, U&E, coagulation screen, and group and save), and prescribe IV fluids. I would consent and mark the patient after explaining the diagnosis and management to the patient.

The anaesthetist and theatre team must also be alerted. Rarely, in some instances, when the diagnosis is unclear, compartment pressures could be measured on the ward. However, more usually, treatment for compartment syndrome is emergency fasciotomy in theatre.

- Probes
  - What further information would you require?
  - Are there any immediate actions to be taken?
  - How would his care be escalated?
- Positive markers
  - Attends to the patient immediately after recognising the risk of compartment syndrome
  - Reviews analgesia received since admission
  - Removes any constricting casts or bandages and elevates the limb
  - Performs pertinent examination
  - Escalates patient care urgently
- Negative markers
  - Does not immediately attend to the patient
  - Does not recognise the risk of compartment syndrome immediately
  - Fails to review analgesia and take back slab off
  - Fails to recognise clinical signs of compartment syndrome – pain on passive stretch
  - Does not escalate patient care

Clinical Scenario 32: Septic Arthritis (Knee)

You review a 52-year-old diabetic male with a two-day history of right knee pain in A&E. His knee is swollen, and he struggles to bear weight. He denies any trauma or recent illness but is febrile. How would you approach this patient?

I am concerned that this patient has septic arthritis in his knee. He has a swollen knee, is unable to bear weight, is febrile, and has a risk factor for diabetes. Septic arthritis is an emergency and requires urgent joint washout in theatre, followed by culture-directed IV antibiotics. Another differential is gout. I would attend to this patient urgently.

I would approach this patient using the CCrISP protocol, especially as he could be septic. I would perform an A–E assessment, and excluding any life-threatening injuries, I would focus on the knee. If he is systematically septic, I would start the sepsis 6 – give IV antibiotics, IV fluids, and oxygen; take lactate level and blood cultures; obtain urine output.

I would obtain a complete history that includes recent travel abroad and recent illnesses. I would review his observations, including blood pressure, heart rate, respiratory rate, oxygen saturation, and temperature. Blood glucose monitoring is vital. After providing adequate analgesia, I would then proceed to examine the knee joint. Attention to the presence of effusion, skin changes (erythema, wounds, warmth to touch, or superficial infections, like cellulitis), range of motion (active and passive), and finally ability to bear weight. I would also briefly assess the joint above and below.

Septic arthritis could result in global sepsis and septic shock. I would gain IV access, obtain initial blood tests (FBC, U&E, CRP, ESR, and uric acid), give IV fluids and oxygen if required, and request a knee x-ray.

I would then escalate this patient's care to my registrar. If there are no skin infections, then I think the patient would benefit from aspirating the knee joint using an aseptic technique. Ideally, this aspiration should be performed prior to the administration of antibiotics. I would be keen to do this under the supervision of my registrar. The colour and consistency of the aspirate should be recorded. The aspirate would be sent for cell count, crystals, culture, and gram stain.

If the patient does have septic arthritis, then I would need to prepare him for theatre. I would explain the potential diagnosis and management plan to the patient, keeping him at the centre of care. He would need to be nil my mouth. If able, I would obtain consent and mark the patient. I would need to inform the anaesthetic team and theatre team.

- Probes
  - What are your priorities?
  - What further information do you require?
  - What investigations would you request?
- Positive markers
  - Recognises that septic arthritis is a critical differential diagnosis
  - Requests appropriate blood tests
  - Recognises the importance of blood glucose monitoring in the septic diabetic patient
  - Escalates patient to the orthopaedic registrar appropriately
- Negative markers
  - Fails to recognise the significance of possible septic arthritis
  - Uses inappropriate investigations
  - Does not consider joint aspiration followed by antibiotics according to local guidelines
  - Fails to escalate urgently

Clinical Scenario 33: Limping Child – Septic Hip

You are asked to review a seven-year-old boy with pain in his right thigh and knee in A&E. He has had a viral illness over the last few days and has been febrile today (38.1°C). The parents have noticed a sudden right-sided limp yesterday. He has previously been fit and well and gives no history of trauma. Outline your approach to this patient.

I am concerned that this patient has septic arthritis of his knee or hip. He has atraumatic right leg pain, is unable to bear weight, is febrile and had a recent illness. I would review this child urgently.

I would approach this patient using the CCrISP protocol. I would perform an A–E assessment, and excluding any life-threatening injuries, I would focus on the hip.

I would obtain a complete history that elaborates on his recent illness and any vaccinations. I would review his observations, including blood pressure, heart rate, respiratory rate, oxygen saturation, and temperature. I would examine the oral cavity, tonsils, and chest. After providing adequate analgesia, I would examine the entire right limb, including the hip, thigh, knee, shin, ankle, and foot. I would pay attention to the resting position of the hip at flexion, abduction, and external rotation to find which position is most comfortable to the patient. I would note the presence of an effusion or swelling, skin changes (erythema, wounds, warmth to touch or superficial infections like cellulitis), range of motion (active and passive), and finally ability to bear weight. I would also briefly assess the pelvis and lumbar spine.

I would gain IV access, obtain initial blood tests (FBC, U&E, CRP, and ESR), give IV fluids, give oxygen if required, and request hip, femur, and knee x-rays.

I would then escalate this patient to my registrar for urgent review. Further investigations could include US scan, MRI scan, or joint aspirate. Septic arthritis is an emergency and requires urgent joint washout in theatre, followed by culture-directed IV antibiotics. Transient synovitis (irritable hip) is a less severe differential diagnosis in a limping child. Depending on our findings, the patient might need to go to theatre, and I would inform the anaesthetic and theatre teams.

I would explain the potential diagnosis and management plan to the family. Dealing with a sick child could be very stressful, I would ensure that I speak to both the child and the parents in a way that they understand.

- Probes
  - What are your priorities?
  - How would examine this patient?
  - How would you further investigate this patient?
  - How would you escalate this patient's care?
- Positive markers
  - Considers the hip joint as the source of the pathology
  - Recognises that septic arthritis is a potentially serious differential diagnosis

- Investigates with appropriate blood tests like FBC, CRP, and ESR
- Escalates to the registrar appropriately
- Negative markers
  - Does not consider the hip joint as the source of pathology
  - Does not consider septic arthritis as a serious differential diagnosis
  - Uses inappropriate examination and investigation
  - Does not escalate appropriately

Cardiothoracic

Clinical Scenario 34: Tension Pneumothorax

You are asked to assess a day 1 post-op 52-year-old man in the thoracic ward. The patient had a right lung volume reduction surgery without intraoperative complications noted. He is complaining of sudden sharp chest pain and shortness of breath. His systolic blood pressure is 80 mm Hg, and his heart rate is 120 bpm. How would you approach this patient?

I am concerned that this patient has tension pneumothorax and he is developing an obstructive type of shock secondary to mediastinal shifting. I would attend to this patient immediately without delay and would activate the peri-arrest call. I would inform and escalate to my registrar as soon as possible.

I would approach the patient using the CCrISP protocol. I would assess his airway by first speaking to him. I would ensure he is on high-flow oxygen with a target oxygen saturation of close to 100% (unless the patient is at risk of hypercapnic [type II] respiratory failure). If he responds, I would move on to assess his breathing. I would look for bilateral chest rise, bilateral chest sounds, and a central trachea. At this stage, if I hear unilateral breath sounds and feel a shifted trachea, I would be concerned about a tension pneumothorax. I would immediately decompress the patient using a large-bore cannula in the fifth intercostal space, mid-axillary line, according to the latest ATLS guidelines. I would expect to hear a hiss and an improvement in the patient's condition. I would arrange to set up a chest drain procedure, keeping in mind to inform the rest of the nursing staff to make the preparation more efficient. I would then reassess the patient, starting at A again.

In terms of circulation, I would assess the patient's heart rate, blood pressure, and capillary refill time. I would ensure that bilateral large-bore access is gained. At the same time, I would take blood specimens for blood gas, full blood count, U&E, LFTs, clotting profile, and cross-match. For disability, I would calculate his GCS and obtain his temperature and blood glucose. I would also quickly expose the rest of the extremities to assess.

At this point, I would also review the patient's notes, his operative record, and any chest drain output that he might have. I would then escalate promptly to my registrar or consultant. The patient would need a definitive chest tube placed at the bedside. This would be inserted in the fifth intercostal space, mid-axillary line, using a sterile technique. I would infiltrate the area with a local anaesthetic, cut down 'above the rib below', and puncture the pleural with a blunt instrument. I would then guide the chest drain superiorly and secure it with a 0-silk and air-tight dressing. I would also need to discuss whether the patient needs to return to theatre to close an air leak. If this were the case, I would need to inform the anaesthetic team, nursing, and theatres. Since the peri-arrest team is also likely to be present, I would direct them to perform certain aspects of the resuscitation, such as taking blood gas or requesting a portable chest x-ray.

Throughout all this, I am conscious that this is a highly stressful situation for the patient and his family, and I would attempt to keep them at the centre of care by clearly explaining to them the situation and necessary life-saving treatment for such a condition.

- Probes
  - What are your priorities?
  - What other information would you gather?
  - Which investigations should be done, and immediate management should be anticipated?
  - How would you escalate this patient's care?
  - Where and how would you insert a chest drain?
- Positive markers
  - Recognises that this is a surgical emergency which needs immediate surgical management
  - Recognises that this requires a team-based approach
  - Assesses the patient with a structured A–E approach
  - Anticipates the immediate life-saving management
  - Escalates to the registrar or consultant appropriately
- Negative markers
  - Does not attend immediately and recognise the situation as a surgical emergency
  - Fails to include other members of the surgical team (anaesthetists, theatre nurses, etc.)
  - Uses an unstructured approach to patient assessment
  - Fails to anticipate immediate management
  - Does not escalate patient care appropriately

Clinical Scenario 35: Haemothorax

You are the core surgical trainee on cardiothoracics. During the ward round, you notice that the chest drain of a 52-year-old female patient, day 1 post–left upper lobectomy, is draining frankly bloody output of 500 ml for the past two hours. She is hypotensive and tachycardic. How would you approach this patient?

I am concerned that this patient has hypovolemic shock secondary to a haemothorax. She would likely need to return to theatre. I would attend to this patient immediately. I would inform and escalate to my registrar and consultant as soon as possible. I would activate the major haemorrhage protocol.

I would approach the patient using the CCrISP protocol. I would assess her airway by first speaking to her. I would ensure she is on high-flow oxygen. If she responds, I would move on to assess her breathing. I would look for bilateral chest rising, bilateral chest sounds and a central trachea. I would expect to hear decreased breath sounds and dullness to percussion on the side of the chest drain. For circulation, I would assess the patient's heart rate, blood pressure, and capillary refill time. I would ensure that bilateral large-bore access is gained. At the same time, I would take blood specimens for blood gas, full blood count, U&E, LFTs, clotting profile, and cross-match for four units. I would start 1 litre of warmed crystalloids stat and have a low threshold to start O-negative blood if the patient continues to be hypotensive and tachycardic. For disability, I would calculate her GCS and obtain her temperature and blood glucose. I would then expose her to look at the rest of her extremities to assess.

I would then review the most recent notes, in particular the operative note. I do not think any further investigations, such as a chest x-ray or CT chest, would be of value in this scenario.

After discussing with my registrar and consultant, I would immediately inform the rest of the theatre team, anaesthetist, nursing team, and porters in preparation for an emergency thoracotomy in theatre. During the interim, I would continuously reassess the patient and make sure that haemodynamic stability is achieved by blood transfusion and correction of coagulopathy if present.

Throughout all this, I am conscious that this is a highly stressful situation for the patient and her family, and I would attempt to keep them at the centre of care by involving them in our decision-making.

- Probes
  - What are your priorities?
  - What other information would you gather?
  - Which investigations should be done, and what immediate management should be anticipated?

- How would you escalate this patient's care?
- Positive markers
  - Recognises that the patient is actively bleeding and this is a surgical emergency which needs immediate surgical intervention (thoracotomy)
  - Recognises that this requires a team-based approach
  - Assesses the patient with a structured A–E approach
  - Requests appropriate investigations (e.g. group and screen, FBC, coagulation panel) and anticipates the need for immediate blood transfusion and correcting pre-existing coagulopathy
  - Escalates to the registrar or consultant appropriately
- Negative markers
  - Does not attend immediately and recognise the situation as a surgical emergency
  - Fails to include other members of the surgical team (anaesthetists, theatre nurses, etc.)
  - Uses an unstructured approach to patient assessment
  - Fails to arrange appropriate investigations, secure group and screen, coagulation panel, etc. and anticipate immediate management
  - Does not anticipate the need for immediate blood transfusion and correcting pre-existing coagulopathy
  - Does not escalate patient care appropriately

Clinical Scenario 36: Aortic Dissection

You are on night shift at the ward and was asked by the nurse-in-charge to assess a day 3 post-op CABG patient. The patient is a 62-year-old male, complaining of dizziness, shortness of breath, and sudden severe, sharp pain in the chest and upper back described as 'ripping'. He is hypotensive with a rapid weak pulse. How would you approach this patient?

I am concerned that this patient has hypovolemic shock from aortic dissection. I would attend to this patient immediately. I would inform and escalate to the registrar as soon as possible.

I would approach the patient using the CCrISP protocol. I would assess his airway by first speaking to him. I would ensure he is on high-flow oxygen. If he responds, I would move on to assess his breathing. I would look for bilateral chest rising, bilateral chest sounds, and a central trachea. If the airway is intact, I would move on to circulation. I would assess the patient's heart rate, blood pressure, and capillary refill time.

I would ensure that bilateral large-bore access is gained. At the same time, I would take blood specimens for blood gas, FBC, U&E, LFTs, clotting profile, and cross-match for possible blood transfusion. I would start 1 litre of warmed crystalloids stat and have a low threshold to start O-negative blood if the patient continues to be hypotensive and tachycardic. For disability, I would calculate his GCS and obtain his temperature and blood glucose. I would do a cardiovascular exam and examine the patient's central and peripheral pulses.

As I am concerned that this patient has aortic dissection. I would be quick to escalate this to my registrar and consultant. As the patient is hemodynamically unstable, I would arrange to perform transthoracic echocardiography (TTE), which would provide a good overview of the nature of dissection. If the dissection is a type A dissection, then it would necessitate an emergency surgical intervention. I would also consider trans-oesophageal echocardiography (TOE) for definitive diagnosis of acute aortic dissection in addition to the TTE. Depending on the local expertise and availability, this could be performed in ITU or operating theatre to confirm the diagnosis and better evaluate the aortic valve. I would not consider a CT scan as the patient is haemodynamically unstable.

Throughout all these, I would ensure clear communication with the nursing staff, anaesthetists, and theatre teams. I would ensure clear communication with the patient and his family and would keep them at the centre of care by involving them in our decision-making.

- Probes
  - What are your priorities?
  - Which investigations can be done immediately?
  - How would you escalate this patient's care?
- Positive markers
  - Recognises that this is a surgical emergency
  - Assesses the patient with a structured A–E approach
  - Requests appropriate investigations
- Negative markers
  - Does not recognise this is a surgical emergency
  - Requests a CT in an unstable patient
  - Uses an unstructured approach to patient assessment
  - Does not escalate patient care appropriately

Clinical Scenario 37: Atrial Fibrillation with Rapid Ventricular Response

You are asked to see a day 3 post-op tissue aortic valve and mitral valve replacement patient. The patient is a 72-year-old female with light-headedness. Her systolic blood pressure is 100 mm Hg. Telemetry shows no visible P waves and an irregularly irregular rhythm with a heart rate of 140 bpm. How would you approach this patient?

In this scenario, I am concerned that the patient has atrial fibrillation. This patient could develop haemodynamic instability due to ventricular underfilling from rapid ventricular response atrial fibrillation. I would inform and escalate to my registrar and attend to the patient immediately.

I would approach the patient using the CCrISP protocol. I would assess her airway by first speaking to her. I would ensure she is on high-flow oxygen. If she responds, I would move on to assess her breathing. I would look for bilateral chest rising, bilateral chest sounds, and a central trachea. If the airway is intact, I would move on to circulation. I would assess the patient's heart rate, blood pressure, and capillary refill time. I would ensure that bilateral large-bore access is gained.

I would arrange for an urgent ECG. At the same time, I would take blood specimens for blood gas, FBC, U&E, LFTs, clotting profile, thyroid function tests, and cross-match. For disability, I would calculate her GCS and obtain her temperature and blood glucose.

I would start the patient on rate control medications. In a stable patient, I would consider oral therapy, but the intravenous route could also be considered to achieve more rapid rate control. The response to the medication would be assessed via continuous cardiac monitoring.

I would look for common causes of atrial fibrillation, such as electrolyte derangements (e.g. hypokalaemia, hypomagnesemia) and dehydration. I would also check the patient's oral anticoagulation status. Most post-operative cardiac surgery patients are on prophylactic doses of anticoagulation for venous thromboembolism. If this is the case, then necessary dose adjustments (keeping in mind the renal profile and other contraindications) should be made to achieve a therapeutic anticoagulation cover.

As the patient is haemodynamically stable, I would also discuss the case with the anaesthetist, theatre team, and nursing staff in anticipation for a possible DC cardioversion in case the patient becomes haemodynamically unstable.

As atrial fibrillation is the most common arrhythmia after cardiac surgery and is considered benign in a third of patients, I would speak to the patient to explain and reassure her.

- Probes
  - What are your priorities?
  - How would you manage this patient?
  - How would you escalate this patient's care?

- Positive markers
  - Assesses the patient with a structured A–E approach
  - Requests appropriate investigations
  - Escalates to the registrar or consultant appropriately
- Negative markers
  - Uses an unstructured approach to patient assessment
  - Fails to arrange appropriate investigations
  - Does not plan for what happens if the patient becomes unstable

chapter ten

Management Scenarios

William Rea, Saarah Ebrahim, Hari Nageswaran,
Humayun Razzaq, Anokha Oomman Joseph,
and Janso Padickakudi Joseph

Management Scenario 1: Poor Training

You are the core surgical trainee on the cardiothoracic team. There is an extended healthcare team, including advanced nurse practitioners. Your consultant expects you to do all the ward jobs, and you find it difficult to get to theatre. The nurse practitioner gets to theatre regularly and is being trained in vein harvesting. How would you approach this situation?

The main issues in this scenario are the distribution of workload, patient safety, and my training requirements.

First, I want to seek more information. What is my role on the team, and what competencies could I acquire during this rotation? Are there other core surgical trainees in the team and what has their experience been? Are there specific workflows in place which require the nurse practitioner to assist, such as for complex cases? Is vein harvest a skill that is also suitable for core trainees? What other operative exposure is available? Cardiothoracic surgery is a complex multidisciplinary speciality, and I would consider the broader picture and my role within it. However, as a core surgical trainee, it is imperative for me to progress surgically during the rotation.

Patient safety is important in this scenario if the burden of workload is not shared. This could result in patient care being compromised, and therefore, the patient would need to be dealt with as a priority. In a long-term sense, patients might also be harmed if junior doctors do not acquire the basic surgical skills they should have during CST.

I would show initiative by reflecting on why I am finding it difficult to get to theatre. Are there other members of the team on the ward that could help with jobs? Is there anything in particular I am struggling to do? Could I maximise my time in theatre by, for example, doing urgent jobs first and then completing the jobs after my theatre time? I would also

DOI: 10.1201/9781003350422-11

speak to the nurse practitioner in a non-confrontational manner to better understand how they have been able to manage their other commitments with theatre time. In addition, I might find that they are at the end of their learning curve and be ready to teach vein harvest.

I would approach my consultant in a non-confrontational manner and convey my interest in wanting to learn and assist in theatre. I want to show an interest both on and off the ward and share my training needs with the consultant. The consultant might have some reasoning as to why they would like me to do the ward jobs. They might see training opportunities for me outside of vein harvesting.

If I do not feel comfortable discussing with the nurse practitioner or consultant directly, I might discuss this with my registrar, who could encourage my attendance in theatre. I could approach the rota coordinator to ask whether my ward days could be built into my rota and have assigned theatre days.

If my concerns are unresolved, I would escalate them to my trainee representative. If my training is being impacted significantly, I would involve my training program director early. The Royal College tutor, clinical director, and director of medical education might also need to be involved.

I would aim to manage this situation in a calm and professional manner. Finally, I would reflect on how I have approached this situation and perhaps make a reflective entry on my portfolio.

- Probes
  - What are your priorities?
  - What other information could you gather?
  - How could patient safety be compromised?
  - Who else can you involve?
- Positive markers
  - Seeks information proactively
  - Speaks directly to the nurse practitioner
  - Speaks directly to the consultant and shows an interest and willingness to learn
  - Escalates appropriately
  - Has insight into the broader context of the team
- Negative markers
  - Is confrontational
  - Is solely focused on their training needs
  - Escalates rapidly, with incomplete information
  - Does not offer solutions

Management Scenario 2: False Documentation

You are the core surgical trainee on general surgery.
The night SHO hands over a day 1 post-left-hemicolectomy patient, whom she had treated with sedation for agitation overnight. The patient is found to be in haemorrhagic shock on the ward round and is taken back to theatre for an emergency laparotomy.
You notice the night SHO has altered her documentation to state that she had suspected intra-abdominal bleeding and handed this over to you. How would you approach this situation?

My main concerns here are patient safety, probity, and professionalism. Duty of candour also comes into play.

I would want to first seek more information regarding the unwell patient. I could do this by reviewing the notes and the night doctor's documentation, any observational charts, and scans. I would review the operative note to understand what was found during the return to theatre. Patient safety is paramount here, and I would ensure that was a priority in this situation.

I would also consider whether the night doctor is a regular member of staff or a locum doctor. I would want to know if this level of clinical error is a recurrent issue and whether anyone else has raised concerns. I would assess if other unwell patients are at risk of deterioration.

Once patient safety is established, I would speak to the night junior doctor in a non-confrontational manner to understand her version of events. I would state my concern that documentation had been altered. I would enquire whether the night shift was particularly busy, and there might have been other reasons that this unwell patient was mismanaged. The junior doctor might have some personal issues that are clouding her judgement, and in this case, I would try to support and encourage her to seek further help. They might understand that what they have done is unprofessional and might apologise and move to rectify the situation. However, it might be very difficult for me to speak to the night junior doctor directly, and this would require escalation.

Altering documentation is a serious breach of GMC guidelines for acting with honesty and integrity. Given that I am implicated in this situation, I would escalate to my clinical and educational supervisors. I would keep contemporaneous records of all conversations to ensure these are documented properly. This situation needs to be handled formally. The consultant overseeing this patient and the night doctor's supervisor would need to be involved. If necessary, I might want to seek support from bodies such as the BMA or my defence union. This situation would need to be escalated to the clinical director of the surgical department. Support would be required for the night junior doctor, and she might require support from occupational health or further training and education. If a local investigation shows a deliberate alteration of documentation, this would likely result in disciplinary action. The decision for further escalation including to GMC would be made by the consultant and educational supervisor and would be based on the severity of the situation.

Finally, the patient would need to be informed of the delay in diagnosis, applying principles of duty of candour. The patient should receive an apology. It is likely that the consultant in charge would want to lead this discussion, but I would have been keen to contribute. Given the gravity of the situation, I would reflect on my actions and consider a reflective portfolio entry.

- Probes
  - What are your priorities?
  - What other information could you gather?
  - Who else can you involve?
- Positive markers
  - Considers patient safety as a priority
  - Understands the gravity of altering documentation
  - Escalates appropriately
  - Documents conversations
  - Considers duty of candour
- Negative markers
  - Does not address professionalism
  - Does not address patient safety
  - Does not address the duty of candour
  - Discusses the situation with other colleagues, resulting in a hostile environment
  - Is defensive and/or confrontational

Management Scenario 3: Never Event

You are the core surgical trainee on the colorectal team. You take a patient to theatre for persistent discharge from a perianal abscess wound that has been going on for months. You find a retained tonsil swab deep within the abscess cavity. How would you approach this situation?

A retained swab is a never event. The other issues here are patient safety, duty of candour, and organisational learning.

Patient safety is paramount in this scenario. I would address the clinical situation, remove the tonsil swab, and debride the cavity as required.

Intra-operatively, I would escalate this to my registrar or consultant so that they could also attend and assess the situation. I would meticulously document my findings in an operative report and ensure that it is countersigned by a senior.

In the first instance, the patient would need to be informed once they are out of surgery. Given the seriousness of the situation as a core trainee, I would speak to the patient along with the consultant in charge of the patient's care. The patient would need to be informed of the intra-operative findings and the management going forward. Per duty of candour guidelines from the GMC, I would apologise on behalf of the team and explain what steps we would be taking to investigate this further and give them information if they wish to speak to PALS. I would document the conversation with them in the notes.

I would enter a Datix for this never event. This event would require a full investigation under NHS England's Serious Incident Framework. The organisation should engage in learning from this event, and the findings of the investigation should be presented at the clinical governance meeting, with all relevant stakeholders. It should also be determined who the surgeon was at the index operation. The surgeon would need to be informed by a more senior member of the team. A review of the previous surgery would need to be performed to understand the events that led to this never event.

The WHO checklist is in place to prevent situations like this from arising, and therefore, the error in this process would need to be determined in the investigation of the incident to prevent it from happening again.

The surgeon who performed the operation should be advised to speak to their supervisor, as well as the BMA and their defence union. I would reflect on what other measures could be put in place to prevent this from happening again, such as more education of staff about following correct protocols.

- Probes
  - What are your priorities?
  - What other information could you gather?
  - Who else can you involve?
  - How should this be discussed with the patient?
  - How will this information be relayed appropriately to the rest of the team?
- Positive markers
  - Deals with patient safety as their first priority
  - Is meticulous in their documentation
  - Considers duty of candour
  - Appreciates the gravity of the situation
  - Identifies this as a never event

- Negative markers
  - Does not deal with patient safety first
  - Does not escalate intra-operatively
  - Does not document meticulously
  - Does not raise a Datix
  - Does not recognise the never event
  - Does not consider organisational learning
  - Appoints individual blame

Management Scenario 4: Managing Juniors

You are the core surgical trainee on the urology team. Your FY1 comes to work late almost all days of the week. How would you approach this situation?

My main concerns from the outset are patient safety, professionalism, and support for my colleague.

Patient safety could be compromised if the FY1's lateness is causing others to pick up the workload. The FY1 might miss out on handover at the start of the day, and this might compromise clinical care. Patient safety should be a priority throughout, and I would first and foremost ensure that there is adequate coverage to take care of patients.

I would want to establish if there is a reason for the FY1 coming late to work. I would speak to my FY1 in a non-confrontational manner and understand their perspective.

I would ensure they are aware of when their shift starts. In a supportive manner, I would try to find out if there are any underlying issues preventing good timekeeping. I would find out if the FY1 is undergoing personal problems that might be causing them to be late to work.

If there are extenuating circumstances such as caring responsibilities or health-related issues, I would work with the FY1 to determine how I could support them. The team would need to consider what measures could be put in place to ensure patient safety and the FY1's professional success. This might require the input of occupational health, the rota coordinator, the consultants in the department, the FY1's educational/clinical supervisors, and the foundation programme training director.

If there are not any extenuating circumstances, I would explain to them the importance of turning up to work on time. I would then review the situation over a period to see if there has been any change, trying to address this informally.

If there are no extenuating circumstances and the FY1 does not change their behaviour, I would escalate this to their educational supervisor. This is an issue of professionalism and might have to be dealt with formally. It might need to be escalated to the foundation programme training director.

If there is a significant breach of professionalism that could not be dealt with at a local level, it might require escalation, even to the GMC. I understand that this type of escalation could be very stressful for the FY1, and I would ensure that they are supported and not vilified throughout this process.

Given the sensitive nature of the situation, I would reflect on my actions and consider a reflective portfolio entry.

- Probes
  - What are your priorities?
  - What other information could you gather?
  - How could patient safety be compromised?
  - Who else can you involve?
- Positive markers
  - Approaches the FY1 directly
  - Considers patient safety
  - Is aware of the support networks in place for the junior doctor
  - Is non-judgmental
- Negative markers
  - Escalates quickly, without full information
  - Avoids speaking to the FY1
  - Does not consider alternative reasons for lateness

Management Scenario 5: Conflict with Senior

You are the core surgical trainee in urology. The registrar in your firm is abrupt and makes you feel unwelcome in theatres. What would you do?

This is an unfortunate and far from ideal situation. The main issues here are professionalism, potential bullying, and the impact this could have on teamwork.

Once I have realised that this is consistent behaviour from the registrar, I would find a suitable time and place to talk to them. I would try to be careful and concise with my words when telling them how their behaviour makes me feel, and at the same time, I would ask what is making them behave like this. I would explain to them that this situation is making it very difficult for me to achieve the most out of this placement in terms of clinical skills and theatre opportunities, which is detrimental to my training. I would explain that this kind of behaviour makes me feel unwelcome in my own workplace. Whilst having this conversation, I would keep an open mind to what they have to say and whether or not there are any concerns from their side. For example, they might be concerned with my level of anatomical knowledge or preparation for cases. Based on their response and engagement with the discussion, I would decide on future steps to ensure that this issue gets resolved in a timely and efficient manner. I would make contemporaneous records of our discussion.

I would consider the impact that my relationship with the registrar has on patient safety. If we are working very closely on a team, then we need to be able to discuss things openly. In particular, I would need to be able to ask questions relating to patient care without the fear of being reprimanded. To ensure that patient safety is a priority, I might need to involve my consultant early and escalate concerns directly to them.

I would be mindful of the fact that I could and should discuss such issue with my assigned educational supervisor and clinical supervisor and see what advice they have to offer. They might also be able to take steps to mitigate this situation, such as having a formal or informal meeting with the registrar in question to discuss the issue at hand. I would ensure that I discuss with my AES and CS about protected theatre time, as there would be other theatre opportunities which I could utilise whilst this issue is being resolved. I am aware that any training issues could be raised with the local surgical tutor, who could take the necessary steps to ensure equal opportunities are being provided. If I have concerns about mental health or require further support, I might contact the professional support units or occupational health. If this is significantly impacting my training, I might also speak to my training programme director or the director of medical education.

Finally, the registrar in question might also require support. Their expressions of abruptness might indicate an issue with their personal or professional life. They might have caring responsibilities, health issues, or professional issues that are causing them to react this way. With the correct people involved, hopefully these issues could also be uncovered and addressed, ideally informally at a local level.

- Probes
  - What are your priorities?
  - What other information could you gather?
  - How could patient safety be compromised?
  - Who else can you involve?
- Positive markers
  - Recognises the issues of professionalism and potential bullying
  - Understands that this behaviour is putting their ability to look after patients
  - Realises that this behaviour is negatively affecting their training experience
  - Is aware of escalation pathways and people to escalate to (i.e. TPD/AES/CS)
  - Recognises the need for support for self and registrar

- Negative markers
  - Downplays the situation and behaviour
  - Does not realise the repercussions of such behaviour on training
  - Does not consider escalation
  - Does not seek support

Management Scenario 6: Bullying

You are the core surgical trainee on general surgery. You note that one consultant is rude to another colleague on a routine basis, both in clinics and in theatres. You have witnessed your colleague being screamed at and called names. What would you do?

This is a very undesirable situation with a clear-cut display of bullying on the consultant's part. I would be most concerned about my colleague's mental health and well-being, as well as their ability to concentrate on work and perform day-to-day clinical duties. This is an issue of professionalism, with a likely impact on patient safety.

Initially, I would sit down with the colleague informally. I would inquire what their thoughts are on the matter, whether or not they recognise the bullying, and whether are they aware of their rights and support available. The situation is particularly serious if the colleague is a trainee, as the power differential between consultant and trainee could be intimidating. I would encourage them to discuss the issue with their educational or clinical supervisor as well as their line manager. I would also signpost them to the guardian of freedom to speak up. If the colleague is a trainee, they might wish to involve their trainee representative, Royal College tutor, or training programme director. These behaviours typically follow a pattern and sometimes go unescalated as individuals are not aware of their rights or means to escalate; however, once escalated, this could lead to repercussions for the individual involved. I would be mindful of the mental health impact such situations could have on an individual and would encourage them to seek health from occupational health or their GP, making their own well-being the first priority.

In order to protect patient safety, I would offer to cover them for any clinical work, rota permitting, whilst they work on this issue. I would also volunteer to provide a witness statement, in case this is required for any formal proceeding. I would meanwhile advise them to discuss with the rota manager and clinical lead to not share any clinical commitments with the consultant in question for the time being.

As a core trainee, confronting a consultant about bullying and harassing behaviour might feel very daunting. If I felt able, I would approach this as an informal discussion with the consultant, as they might not be aware of the impact of their words and actions on others.

They might perceive the situation differently. Perhaps they think they are being humorous. However, if I could not speak to the consultant directly, with the permission of my colleague, it might be sensible to involve other consultants in the department or the clinical director. If the concerns are not addressed, this might need to be escalated to the chief medical officer or even the GMC. The consultant themselves might need support as their behaviour might be an expression of difficulties in their personal or professional life.

- Probes
  - What are your priorities?
  - What other information could you gather?
  - How could patient safety be compromised?
  - Who else can you involve?
- Positive markers
  - Recognises bullying
  - Knows the colleague need support
  - Discuss with the colleague
  - Discusses with the consultant
  - Encourages the colleague to report bullying and seek support
- Negative markers
  - Is unable to recognise bullying
  - Does not signpost about the support available to the colleague
  - Downplays the situation
  - Is confrontational
  - Does not take personal responsibility

Management Scenario 7: Clinical Governance

You are the core surgical trainee on the vascular team. A patient has developed a wound infection after a fem-fem bypass. The ward sister states that this patient is under Mr Brown, and all his wounds get infected. How would you approach this situation?

The main issues here are patient safety and teamwork.

My priority is to make sure the patient is being optimally managed and is on appropriate antibiotics based on trust guidelines and recent wound swabs. If they are systemically unwell, they might require specialist management with microbiology. Rarely, they would require surgical re-exploration.

Once the clinical issues are dealt with, I would seek to gather more information. I would speak to the ward sister in private and ask about her concerns regarding the wound infection rate. I would enquire if this has been looked into before, or if it is a new concern. In a non-confrontational manner, I would also speak to my registrar and Mr Brown to see if this aspect of our care is something that would merit an audit to investigate it further.

I want to use my initiative and do two things: raise a Datix and consider an audit or quality improvement project. I would want to raise a Datix as this is an adverse, event and there is potential for organisational learning. Once the team agrees, I would contact the audit department of my hospital to register an audit, looking at the wound infection rate in our wards in comparison to a local or national standard. This would provide the infection rates for Mr Brown and the other surgeons within the unit to indeed see if there is a difference between the different surgeons.

Another way to approach this would be to conduct a quality improvement project. There are multiple stakeholders involved in a patient's pathway. I would want to know if there is a standardised pre-operative pathway that includes antibiotic administration and if this is being complied with. If there is none, then I would speak to my seniors about being involved in designing a clinical process pathway for pre-operative management of patients, including antibiotics at induction. Both an audit and a QUIP could be presented at the morbidity and mortality conference.

There is clearly also a teamwork issue that needs to be addressed, if the sister in charge was concerned about the wound infection rates, she should feel empowered to voice her concerns so that things could be investigated further.

Finally, Mr Brown and his team might require support in order to decrease the wound infection rates for their patients. This might require involvement from multiple stakeholders, including the theatre team, post-operative ward team, and infection control.

- Probes
  - What are your priorities?
  - What other information could you gather?
  - How could patient safety be compromised?
  - Who else can you involve?
- Positive markers
  - Approaches the scenario in a structured manner
  - Escalates appropriately
  - Considers patient safety
  - Appreciates multiple stakeholders
- Negative markers
  - Places blame on a single individual
  - Fails to escalate
  - Does not consider audit or QUIP

Management Scenario 8: Conflict Resolution

*You are the core surgical trainee on the orthopaedic team. You are in theatre
with your registrar who is new to the NHS. Your consultant is in a meeting.
Theatre staff say that the list is overrunning, and the last patient needs to
be cancelled. You and your registrar feel you will be able to finish the case in
time. How would you approach this situation?*

The main issues in the scenario here are patient safety, teamwork, and
professionalism.

The first thing I would do is gather more information. I would take
into account the theatre staff's concerns and why they think the last case
needs to be cancelled. I would also determine the current time and what
time the list is due to finish to establish with the registrar if this is sufficient time to finish. I would like to know if the concern about finishing
late is a perceived issue or a real issue. I would discuss with the anaesthetist what time realistically the patient would be ready to start the operation. I would ask the registrar how long they think the case would take.
I would also take into account the patient-specific details – how urgent
the case is, how long they have been waiting, the impact of not delaying
the operation, and how soon they might be able to be rebooked. I would
consider the surgical team. Whilst the registrar might be new to the NHS,
they might be a very experienced and technically competent surgeon. The
consultant being unavailable is another issue to take into consideration. Is
their meeting urgent? Would they be returning? Could I and the registrar
start the procedure and the consultant join us at a critical stage?

Taking all these factors into consideration, I think it is worth having
a multidisciplinary discussion with the orthopaedic registrar, the theatre
staff, the anaesthetist, and recovery staff. Ideally, the orthopaedic consultant
would also be present for this discussion, but if not, they could potentially
join by phone if they were able to step out from their meeting. Between the
group all those factors could be weighed up and a decision to proceed or
delay the case could be made. We should also consider all other options
apart from cancellation, including potentially using another free theatre
(potentially with another team) or using the emergency list if appropriate.

If the decision is made to cancel the patient, I would apologise to the
patient personally. I would attempt to speak to the booking coordinator to
find a new date before the patient leaves the hospital. I might direct them
to the PALS service.

I need to support my team. If theatre staff want to cancel the case
because of overwork and burnout, then this would need to be dealt with
at a departmental level. If, however, the decision to cancel the case was
routed in underlying bias against a registrar new to the NHS, then this is
a cultural problem that needs addressing.

I would also consider my consultant's professionalism in leaving a new registrar to operate independently. The consultant should not be attending a meeting at the same time as an elective list that is scheduled, unless they are confident of the registrar's abilities and continue to be available throughout the case. If I have concerns over my consultant's professionalism, I might first choose to discuss this with my clinical supervisor. If this is a recurrent issue, then it might need to be escalated further to the clinical director or chief medical officer.

- Probes
  - What are the issues here?
  - What factors would affect the decision whether or not to proceed?
  - What are the implications for the list overrunning?
  - Who bears ultimate responsibility for making the decision?
- Positive markers
  - Approaches scenario in a structured manner
  - Takes into account technical and non-technical aspects of theatre list management
  - Gathers relevant information
- Negative markers
  - Shows an aggressive response to cancelled cases
  - Fails to take a multidisciplinary approach
  - Is unwilling to receive new information

Management Scenario 9: Confidentiality

You are the core surgical trainee on the breast team. One of the departmental secretaries is looking up her daughter's CT scan results. She asks you to interpret the report, which states that there is metastatic breast cancer. How would you approach this situation?

This is a complex issue, involving probity, confidentiality, and professional relationships.

The first thing I would do is sit down with the secretary and ask her if she would like to share what has been happening with her daughter. Clearly, she is concerned and anxious and would certainly be in need of support due to the circumstances. It might be that there has been limited communication between the breast team and the secretary and her daughter so they have questions that I might be able to answer. Hopefully, by gaining an oversight of the situation, I could prevent this from progressing any further.

However, if pressed to provide an interpretation of the CT report, I would politely decline. I would explain that although I could interpret

the report, the implications of the report on the management and treatment are not down to me and would be better discussed in the MDT and
communicated formally by the responsible team. I could offer to contact
the breast MDT coordinator to ensure that the patient is discussed at the
next possible opportunity. I might also alert the consultant responsible for
the patient's care to the fact that a red flag report has been created.

Unfortunately, the secretary's actions are a breach of information
governance policies within the NHS. Therefore, this would need to be
escalated to the secretary's line manager. I would speak to my clinical
supervisor in the first instance to see how to proceed with escalating this.
The patient would also need to be informed, as the information might
have been retrieved without her consent. Depending on the secretary's
manager's view of the situation, this might lead to retraining or disciplinary action.

- Probes
  - What are the issues here?
  - How might you de-escalate the situation?
  - Who should be informed?
- Positive markers
  - Approaches scenario in a sympathetic manner
  - Considers avenues of escalation
  - Considers the emotions of the secretary and her daughter
  - Suggests ways they can help expedite further management
- Negative markers
  - Uses an insensitive approach to speaking to the secretary
  - Shows no effort to support the secretary
  - Reads report and advises the secretary without consideration of
    confidentiality or probity

Management Scenario 10: Showing Initiative

*You are the core surgical trainee on the orthopaedic team. You work with a
sarcoma specialist consultant, who does very complex surgery. You feel like
you are not being allowed to do anything in theatre and your logbook is suffering. How would you approach this situation?*

This is not an uncommon situation, with issues affecting training and
progression and long-term patient safety.

I would start by gathering some further information by reviewing my
logbook and also reviewing my actions in each recorded operation. It might
then be worth comparing my logbook to other core surgical trainees in the
department to see if they are facing similar issues or if they are getting more

practical operative experience. I would assess if I had operative experience elsewhere, in other lists, or if this is my only time in theatre.

Patient safety is relevant here for the future as a direct consequence of training. If junior surgeons are not trained well at an early stage, their higher training would be more complicated and might ultimately result in a less well-trained operative surgeon at the end of their training.

Once I have collected the data, I would discuss the findings with my consultant, especially if my operative logbook is significantly less extensive than other trainees within the department. But I would be proactive about making suggestions to remedy the situation. Whilst it would not be appropriate for a junior trainee to be taking on whole complex operations, there would be parts of the operation it would be reasonable to expect the trainee to accomplish under senior supervision. Whilst the dissection and resection might not be suitable for a core trainee, prepping, draping, initial incision, and approach, and then closure might be reasonable to complete unless there are patient-specific issues. I would come to the cases prepared, having read up about the patient, the relevant anatomy, and the procedure. Another suggestion might be to request swapping the occasional operating list with other trainees, allowing them the opportunity to see complex sarcoma surgery whilst I assist and learn from other surgeons with other subspeciality interests. I would work with the rota coordinator to facilitate this.

If my suggestions are turned down or not acted upon, then I would escalate this to my educational supervisor. If still there is no improvement in my operative exposure, I might involve the director of medication education, my trainee representative, and training programme director. The Royal College tutor at my hospital should also be aware.

- Probes
  - What are the issues here?
  - How could you broach this topic with your consultant?
  - What constructive suggestions could you make to aid your training?
- Positive markers
  - Approaches scenario in a sympathetic manner
  - Is non-confrontational
  - Has constructive suggestions for ways to improve training
  - Considers routes of escalation in the event of no change
- Negative markers
  - Escalates inappropriately
  - Accepts the status quo
  - Is confrontational

Management Scenario 11: Negotiating Skills

You are the core surgical trainee on the ENT team. You are assisting your consultant on a head and neck list. He leaves you to close the large neck wound. When the consultant leaves theatre, the staff start complaining among themselves. You hear them say that you are operating too slowly and they want to leave on time. How would you approach this situation?

This is a tricky situation involving multi-professional communication, training requirements, and a balance with service need.

I would start by apologising that they felt I am operating slowly, but I would say that I am doing what I feel is safest for the patient and that rushing would likely lead to a mistake, ultimately taking an even longer time. I would also stress that this is the best way for me to learn and that by allowing me to proceed, I would be faster and more precise in the future. I would avoid mentioning that comments about my speed of operating are only likely to slow me down further and that surgical speed is only one marker of technical excellence. I would also consider whether closing a large neck wound is truly within my competence and whether I do, in fact, need help to close it appropriately and in time.

I would acknowledge theatre staff's need to leave on time, as their time is of value. Theatre staff should not feel overworked and burdened. I would make the suggestion that I might proceed undisturbed for the next 15 minutes. If I am not making progress, then I would suggest that we call either a registrar or the consultant back in to help. If this suggestion is accepted, then I would proceed to finish the case.

Following this, I would reflect on the case and my technical progress throughout my training. If I feel that I am still operating slowly, then I might look into getting further practice, either in theatre or on simulated tissues. I could find some expired sutures to take home to practice my hand ties and other technical skills to improve my confidence and surgical fluency. I would also discuss with any colleagues if they experienced similar comments and, if so, how they approached the situation. Comparing actions and outcomes could help if I were to encounter a similar situation in the future. I would also debrief the case with my consultant and enquire why they felt they could entrust me with this closure and take on any feedback.

Finally, I would consider whether the episode in theatre was a micro-aggression against me. I would consider whether this is a recurring theme. If the culture in theatres is not conducive to training, then I would discuss this with my educational supervisor. We might need to involve other stakeholders, such as the theatre coordinator or theatre team lead, to see how this could be remedied in the future.

- Probes
  - What are the issues here?
  - What other information could you gather?
  - How could patient safety be compromised?
  - Who else can you involve?
- Positive markers
  - Approaches scenario in a thoughtful manner
  - Considers multiple sources of feedback
  - Considers methods of self-improvement
- Negative markers
  - Does nothing
  - Becomes confrontational
  - Shows no reflection on personal performance

Management Scenario 12: Dealing with Racism

You are the core surgical trainee. A patient tells you they want to see a doctor of a different ethnicity than your own. They get abusive when you try to reason with them. How would you proceed?

The behaviour of this patient is an example of racism and should not be accepted. Despite trying to reason with the patient, they have become abusive, and therefore, it is no longer appropriate for me to carry on treating them. I would stay calm, stop engaging with the patient, and remove myself from their immediate environment.

How I proceed next would depend on the clinical circumstances. If the patient requires emergency treatment, I would request the nearest available suitable doctor to take over their care, ideally someone more senior than me. Although ill health is not a valid excuse for racist behaviour, it could be a contributing factor causing delirium. The patient should still have emergency treatment.

If, however, they do not need urgent care, usually hospital policy suggests a zero-tolerance approach to abuse against staff. I would escalate this incident to my registrar, my consultant, and the ward manager. It should be explained to the patient that their behaviour is unacceptable, and they could not discriminate healthcare staff for their background. The patient should be told to change their behaviour.

According to the patient's level of abuse and whether it is verbal or physical, it might be necessary to call either hospital security or the police. My primary concern would be to make the environment safe for myself and others who might require that the patient be moved to another location. If the patient continues to be abusive, senior hospital management might refuse to provide care.

I would also clearly document in the patient's notes exactly what was said by the patient and the circumstances surrounding it. I would also record the names and contact details of those who witnessed or were involved in the incident in case further investigation or evidence is needed in the future. I would then complete a Datix form to record the incident.

Finally, I would consider the impact this has on my well-being. I would discuss this with my consultant and my educational supervisor and ask for further support if required. I am aware that staff support through occupational health or from the BMA is available and that I should seek this if I feel my ability to provide patient care and my medical career are going to be affected by this incident.

- Probes
  - Who could you ask for help?
  - Would you report this behaviour to anyone?
  - What documentation do you need to carry out?
- Positive markers
  - Clearly states this is not acceptable behaviour
  - Calls for assistance early
  - Acknowledges there may be clinical reasons behind the patient's behaviour
  - Remains calm
  - Knows trust policy on racism and abusive behaviour
- Negative markers
  - Argues with patient
  - Ignores racist behaviour of patient and does not report it
  - Fails to obtain help and protect themselves

Management Scenario 13: Rota Cover

You are the core surgical trainee on-call for the day and have finished a 12-hour shift. The night CST has called in sick. How would you approach this situation?

In this situation, my overarching concern is patient safety. I would also consider the workload for the surgical staff.

I would first seek to understand the situation completely. I would see how many patients are left to be seen, how many require urgent intervention, and how many are unwell. I would assess who the night team consists of. Is there an FY1 and a registrar?

I would take the initiative to try and make the situation better. The team should consider all options. There might be a ward FY1 available on nights who might be able to cover some aspects of the on-call team's work. There might be an individual available on short notice to cover the shift.

There might be junior doctors in different specialities who might be able to cross-cover.

I would escalate this situation to the site manager and the consultant on-call. They might be able to help with staffing issues. In particular, the site manager might be able to identify an individual elsewhere in the hospital who might be able to help with specific duties. The site manager or consultant might be able to source a last-minute locum doctor. I would also escalate this to the nurse in charge for admissions, advising that there might be a delay in seeing patients. The nurse in charge and their staff might be able to support the team with ancillary duties, such as taking blood specimens, placing cannulas, or inserting urinary catheters, depending on skill mix.

If no replacement SHO could be found, it would be the responsibility of the registrar on-call to cover the duties, with support from the consultant as required. If it is particularly busy, the consultant might need to come in. Although I would not be required to continue working the night shift, if I am feeling able and capable to do so, I could support my colleagues by staying on for a short period of time to help complete any urgent clinical care that is necessary. However, I would be careful not to provide clinical care when overly tired, and it might be necessary for me to have a rest period before doing so. I think it is important to be a team player and help the night team in any way I could in a difficult situation. However, I would not want to place patients in potential harm by working outside my limitations.

Finally, the rota coordinator needs to be informed the next morning to make sure that there is adequate staffing for the next night shift. If uncovered shifts are a regular occurrence in the department, then I would raise this with my clinical supervisor for further escalation.

- Probes
  - What are the issues here?
  - What other information could you gather?
  - How could patient safety be compromised?
  - Who else can you involve?
- Positive markers
  - Recognises possible harm to patient care and prioritises this
  - Informs the site manager and on-call consultant
  - Attempts to help with finding cover
  - Negotiates to find a solution and offers some level of help
  - Understands the trust policy on requirements for cover in case of absence
- Negative markers
  - Does not help to find a solution
  - Does not escalate to the line manager or consultant
  - Agrees to stay on and cover the duty despite being tired

Management Scenario 14: Breach of Confidentiality

You are the core surgical trainee. You walk into the handover room and find your registrar looking at the medical notes of a patient who is admitted under a different speciality. How would you approach this situation?

I would be concerned here about a possible breach of patient confidentiality. The other issues here are professionalism and the duty of candour.

First, I would approach the registrar and politely enquire about their reason for accessing the notes. They might have a valid reason for doing so, such as providing patient care. However, if they do not have a valid reason, I would remind them of their professional obligation to maintain patient confidentiality.

If the registrar accessed the notes inappropriately, this is a breach of the GMC ethical guidance on confidentiality. As this is an issue of professionalism, unfortunately, I would need to escalate this to their educational supervisor. Although it is possible that this could be resolved at a local level, depending on the severity of the breach, this might lead to disciplinary action. The clinical director, chief medical officer, and training programme director might become involved. The educational supervisor would lead this.

The patient would also need to be told that there has been a breach of their confidentiality. This needs to be disclosed using the duty of candour. The patient should be offered an apology and signposted to the PALS service. It is likely that this disclosure comes best from the consultant in charge of the patient's care.

The registrar involved would require support in this scenario, as it is likely to be stressful. Although I would probably not be best placed to offer the support, occupational health, the registrar's defence union, or the BMA might be good starting points.

I would also reflect in my portfolio about my actions, which are likely to have a significant impact on a colleague. The episode might also make team working with the registrar difficult, and I would need to employ diplomacy and conflict resolution to ensure that the team could provide good clinical care. In such a situation, it might be necessary to separate the two of us on the team, and I would coordinate this with the permission of my educational supervisor and the rota coordinator.

- Probes
  - What are your concerns about this scenario?
  - What reasons might the doctor have for looking in the medical notes?
  - Whom would you inform about the registrar's actions?

- Positive markers
  - Understands there might be a breach of patient confidentiality
  - Takes initiative in establishing whether the registrar has a valid reason
  - Escalates appropriately
  - Knows trust policy on breach of confidentiality
- Negative markers
  - Ignores what they have seen
  - Accepts the registrar's explanation and does not confirm it through other sources
  - Confronts the doctor/becomes angry

Management Scenario 15: Workforce Planning

You are a CST in orthopaedics. You note that there is regular overbooking of clinics. The service manager regularly pulls you from theatres to cover these. You are expected to see patients independently in these clinics with little senior support. How would you approach this situation?

My concerns in this scenario are poor workforce planning, impact on patient safety, and compromised surgical training.

If I am being asked to see patients without sufficient senior supervision, this compromises patient care. If this is happening on a regular basis and I am being reassigned from other activities, including from theatre, my surgical training is being affected.

I would try and find out why this keeps happening by speaking with the service manager in case there is a simple problem that needs resolving. There might be a simple misunderstanding; for example, they might have mistaken me for a registrar. I could also discuss the issue with other trainees to see whether its only me that is affected or whether others are facing a similar problem. I would approach the service manager and express my concerns over the overbooking of clinics. I would make clear the impact that being pulled from the operating room is having on my schedule and training. I would also express concern over the lack of supervision. I would offer solutions, such as increasing staffing levels and rescheduling appointments to reduce the number of overbooked clinics. If there is a solution where we, as trainees, could be better allocated to cover these clinics so that we are not losing learning opportunities and all of us are sharing the workload from clinics evenly, I would be happy to help organise and manage this. For example, I could work with the service manager to create a suitable rota for the clinics. It is important to conduct this conversation in a respectful and professional manner to find a mutually beneficial solution.

I would raise the issue with my educational supervisor. I would review my logbook with them and make sure that I am getting adequate experience. I would also need to involve my training programme director in this instance as service priorities are disrupting my training on a regular basis. There might be other individuals (e.g. trust doctors or registrars) who might be able to cover some clinics. The Royal College tutor would also need to be informed.

- Probes
  - What issues are you concerned about?
  - What information could you gather to support your case?
  - Who would you discuss this with?
  - Who could you escalate this to?
- Positive markers
  - Acknowledges this is a management issue
  - Recognises patient care is at risk
  - Recognises training provision is inadequate
  - Acknowledges their own limitations
  - Discusses with others to gather information and data
  - Takes initiative in finding a solution
  - Knows the structure for escalation within hospital trust and deanery
- Negative markers
  - Does not discuss with other trainees and consultants
  - Agrees to manage clinics without supervision
  - Refuses to attend the clinic

Management Scenario 16: Drunk Registrar

You are the core surgical trainee on-call. You can smell alcohol on your registrar's breath. How would you proceed?

I am concerned here about my registrar's ability to provide safe clinical care. Patient safety is potentially at risk. Second, there is an issue of professionalism that needs to be dealt with.

I would approach this sensitive situation cautiously. If I feel comfortable doing so, I would approach the registrar directly. I would speak to them in a private space and express my concerns about alcohol on their breath. I would remind them of their professional responsibilities. I might ask another medical or nursing colleague to witness the conversation.

If the registrar is not receptive to my concerns or if I do not feel comfortable addressing the issue directly, I would escalate this to the consultant. The consultant should advise the registrar to remove themselves from clinical activities and go home for the day to fully recover. I would make sure they have a safe way of getting home and would offer to arrange transport if needed.

The rest of the on-call shift would need covering, and so I would also inform the rota coordinator that a replacement registrar needs to be found as they had to leave for personal reasons. Any patients already seen by the registrar would need a second review to ensure the correct decisions were made.

It is possible this is just an isolated incident. The registrar's educational supervisor would need to be informed. However, since this is a serious breach of professionalism, this is likely to lead to some form of disciplinary action. The chief medical officer or training programme director for the registrar might need to be involved.

The registrar involved would require support in this scenario, as it is likely to be stressful. Although I would probably not be best placed to offer the support, occupational health, the registrar's defence union, or the BMA might be good starting points.

I would also reflect in my portfolio about my actions, which are likely to have a significant impact on a colleague. The episode might also make team working with the registrar difficult, and I would need to employ diplomacy and conflict resolution to ensure that the team could provide good clinical care. In such a situation, it might be necessary to separate the two of us on the team, and I would coordinate this with the permission of my educational supervisor and the rota coordinator.

- Probes
  - How would you approach the discussion with your registrar?
  - What other information would you gather?
  - How would you report this issue?
  - Whom would you escalate this to?
- Positive markers
  - Prioritises patient safety
  - Takes steps to ensure appropriate cover is arranged
  - Reports the incident appropriately
  - Considers possible underlying reasons for colleague's behaviour
- Negative markers
  - Ignores clinical danger
  - Does not report the incident
  - Does not consider the colleague's well-being

chapter eleven

Post-Interview Job Preferencing

Stefanos Gkaliamoutsas and Alex Meredith-Hardy

Preferencing Core Surgical Training (CST) programme posts happens after interviews. You will be contacted via Oriel to submit your preferences. Ranking is an arduous task, as you have to preference hundreds of individual jobs. Some jobs may be run-through training in a certain speciality (these are currently rare). Other jobs may have a specific subspeciality theme. Most jobs are a good mix of various surgical specialities. Unfortunately, there is no good way currently to find out about the different rotations. Be creative and use your network. You can gain valuable insights by speaking to former medical school colleagues, junior doctors, registrars, and consultants about their experiences in different regions.

Questions to Ask Yourself

Some of the questions you may wish to consider when preferencing are as follows:

- Within which speciality will you be aiming to apply for an ST3 number in two years' time?
- How much experience do you need in that speciality to maximise your ST3 application points?
- Do you risk spending too much time in your preferred speciality and therefore losing points on your ST3 application?
- How much experience, if any, do you require within allied specialities for the ST3 programme that you intend on applying to?
- Where do you want to live for the next two years?
- Are there any specialities that you are unwilling to work in?

Reflecting on Your Priorities

Every individual will have different priorities when it comes to preferencing jobs. Some individuals may have a specific place they want to work in and will not consider jobs outside this geographic area. Others may be

DOI: 10.1201/9781003350422-12

determined to get a themed job within their speciality of interest, as this will give you more exposure to this speciality and will therefore prioritise this over location. Approach this period of reflection with a growth mindset, understanding that getting a coveted CST post is more important than the exact configuration of rotations. Unexpected opportunities and experiences may be gained if you are adventurous and geographically mobile.

Ranking Strategy

The key to ranking is to list every single job that you would potentially accept within the first iteration of preferencing. We cannot emphasise this point enough. The first iteration is your best chance to gain a CST post. If you change your mind about which jobs you would accept after the first iteration, you may miss out on hundreds of jobs that you could have potentially secured in subsequent rounds. Rank geographically widely and surgically broadly. We would recommend ranking all run-through jobs first if you are geographically flexible, followed by speciality-themed jobs (if you have a preference).

For individuals aiming to get a job in a themed track, we would advise ranking all these jobs at the top of your list. For example, a trainee wishing to pursue a career in urology should rank urology-themed programmes first. These themselves can be differentiated based on location or preference of the non-urology rotations within that programme. Then the trainee would rank all remaining jobs they would be willing to accept.

For individuals for whom geography is the most important factor, we again recommend preferencing as broadly as possible. Candidates often make the mistake of only ranking a small number of jobs in the first iteration, only realising their mistake when they do not receive an offer. If you are geographically limited, rank the jobs in your deanery of preference and at least two or three surrounding deaneries. You can always hold or reject these job offers later if they really do not fit your life.

Offers Process

All posts that you would be happy to accept should be dragged and dropped into the preferences column. All posts that you would not consider should be put into the 'not wanted' section. Regularly save your preferencing on Oriel as it can time out and you might lose everything that you have done. The preferences are then submitted.

Do not worry if you do not get offered a job in the first round. There is a long process of candidates accepting and rejecting jobs, and there are chances are that you might be offered a post later.

Top Three Tips for Post-Interview Job Preferencing

1. Rank every single job that you would potentially accept within the first iteration of preferencing.
2. Reflect on your priorities of exposure to speciality versus geographic location.
3. Have a growth mindset. Be open-minded about jobs to maximise your chances of getting a national training number.

chapter twelve

Life as a Core Surgical Trainee

Haseem Raja and Janso Padickakudi Joseph

Core surgical training (CST) offers a wealth of opportunities for the budding surgical trainee. It is a time to grow in your clinical skill and knowledge while working in the hospital. It also requires significant commitment outside your clinical work to grow personally and professionally. Whilst the provision of opportunities may differ amongst hospitals and training programmes, it is incumbent upon you to be proactive with your learning and seek out opportunities. Asking for advice and support from seniors will help you navigate the process more smoothly. The biggest challenge, perhaps, is striking a healthy balance between work and life outside of CST, so this requires careful attention.

As you progress through CST, you should consider the following four priorities.

Developing Surgical Skills

First and foremost, CST is about laying the foundation for your surgical skills. You will have the opportunity to rotate through various specialties and develop a broad array of skills. You should approach this with a growth mindset, trying to find opportunities all around you. Be proactive about getting to theatre as much as possible. However, also recognise the value of learning outside of theatre, such as attending clinics or being on-call; it is here that you will learn about decision-making. You should learn something every day. You should actively seek out feedback on your performance as often as possible and reflect on this. CST is a chance for you to understand the case mix and lifestyle associated with different specialties, so enjoy the exploratory part of this process.

A typical week as a CST is varied, consisting of a mixture of sessions, such as ward cover, on-call, clinics, and theatre. If there is a minor ops list with office-based procedures (e.g. clinic-based endoscopy, lumps and bumps under local anaesthesia), these are excellent learning opportunities for CSTs. Attendance at multidisciplinary team meetings is particularly beneficial for reviewing scans and observing how cases are managed.

DOI: 10.1201/9781003350422-13

Passing the MRCS Exam

Becoming a member of the Royal College of Surgeons by passing the MRCS examination is a requirement to finish CST. This goal should be prioritised, especially as preparation for the examination will increase your knowledge base for your clinical rotations. There is a multitude of resources available for passing the examination, and further detail can be found in the portfolio chapter of this book. Although there is not an ideal timeline for this, passing both parts of the examination earlier rather than later will then allow you to focus your efforts on developing your clinical skills.

Completing Portfolio Requirements, Both for ARCP and ST3 Applications

At the beginning of CST, you should look at the portfolio requirements for entry into all higher surgical training programmes that you may be considering. Here, the process for portfolio preparation starts anew. You should build on your successes so far and approach developing your portfolio with rigour and advanced planning. You should consider how you can progress some of the projects that you have already started – can a poster you have presented be turned into a paper? Juggling the tasks of scoring as many portfolio points as possible alongside a busy on-call rota means that you need to have excellent time management and prioritisation skills. You should book courses such as CCrISP and ATLS early, as these are often overbooked. You need to be selective about which research projects you take on, and only commit to those that have the potential to be presented or published. This often means being firm and respectful when turning down some interesting research proposals. You should upload your certificates and evidence contemporaneously so that you do not need to scramble before ARCP. You should also use every opportunity to send workplace-based assessments (WBAs) to meet your ARCP requirements.

Achieving a Work-Life Balance

It is essential to achieve a good work-life balance and avoid the risk of burnout. CST can be physically and mentally draining. You should spend regular quality time with friends and family, continue your hobbies (or find new ones), and engage with your communities. Having a support structure outside of work will set you up for success as a CST when the going gets tough.

Top Five Tips – How to Succeed as a Core Surgical Trainee

1. Aim to complete the MRCS exam in your first year of training.
2. Team up with colleagues to complete ARCP/ST3 portfolio requirements.
3. Utilise your study leave allowance and book courses early.
4. Approach rotating through different surgical placements with a growth mindset.
5. Make time for yourself outside of work.

Case Study: Haseem Raja, ENT Registrar (West Midlands)

Life as a core surgical trainee during the COVID-19 pandemic was equally challenging and exciting. Despite being redeployed to the Infectious Diseases Unit for three months and having significantly reduced training opportunities in Core Surgical Training (CST), I adapted quickly to these changes and maximised my learning opportunities. I was in the favourable position of having a national training number in ENT surgery, so I considered myself very fortunate in comparison to my peers.

Based in a large university teaching hospital, my two-year training programme consisted of four six-month placements in upper GI, ENT (twice luckily), and plastic surgery. This breadth of exposure was great for learning and surgical skill acquisition. Providing night cross-cover for urology and vascular surgery during my first year of training further enriched my overall experience.

I prioritised the exam at the beginning of CST and, through starting my preparations early, was able to successfully complete both parts for MRCS (ENT) during my first year. I found the eMRCS question bank particularly helpful for the Part A MCQ examination. Passing the exam early provided me with ample opportunity in my second year of training to focus on improving my skills in theatre and clinic, as well as preparing for life as an ENT registrar.

Rotating through different surgical specialities provided me with an excellent opportunity to develop a whole array of skills. Plastic surgery, my last rotation of core training, in particular, enabled me to hone my basic surgical skills, including tissue handling and wound closure. Whilst keeping an open mind to surgical opportunities, it was important for me to tailor my learning needs to certain areas; my focus was on becoming competent in performing the common ENT index procedures expected of a day 1 registrar. These procedures included adenotonsillectomy, insertion of grommets, and microlaryngoscopy. I also made an active attempt to get involved in all emergency cases relevant to ENT. To supplement this learning, I utilised my study leave allowance to attend craft courses, such as Functional Endoscopic Sinus Surgery and Temporal Bone Dissection.

Whilst I had the security of a national training number in ENT surgery, I was fully aware of the portfolio demands required for ST3 applications as I had prepared to reapply with the view of moving deaneries due to personal circumstances. I booked courses, such as ATLS and APLS, in advance and only committed to research projects with the potential of being published and presented nationally within 12 months.

To achieve an optimal state of productivity with regard to clinical work and completing portfolio requirements, I needed to recharge my batteries periodically with adequate rest and days away from work. I also made a concerted effort of continuing my hobbies of playing football and undertaking fitness training outside of work; this was crucial for my overall well-being.

chapter thirteen

The Challenges of Life as a Core Surgical Trainee

Gargi Pandey and Janso Padickakudi Joseph

Once you get your Core Surgical Training (CST) number, you take a sigh of relief and think, 'It's time for a break'. Unfortunately, not. Higher surgical training (ST3) applications open only a year after starting CST, so the preparation needs to start immediately.

Tough Workload

Make no mistake, becoming a surgeon is tough. Core surgical training can be overwhelming, busy and frustrating. The laundry list of requirements seems endless. You need to juggle the realities of your day job, prepare for your Annual Review of Competency Progression (ARCP) and start collecting portfolio evidence for ST3 applications. For example, for ST3 in ENT to score maximum points, you need nine publications, eight audits, two national or international oral presentations, two regional oral presentations, two poster presentations, postgraduate degrees, and more. It will be impossible to achieve all of this in a single year. You, therefore, need to plan in advance, set realistic goals, work smart, and also make time for yourself for rest and relaxation.

Feeling Out of Depth

You may rotate through specialities during your CST in which you have very little experience. It can be very daunting to start a job with minimal clinical induction. Often you are thrust into the deep end, especially while on-call. You may find yourself in a situation where you are expected to give specialist advice but feel out of your depth. In this situation, it is important to be proactive, creative, and aware of your own limitations. Overcoming this feeling will take preparation on your part. Read broadly. When you encounter a new case, spend ten minutes to read about the disease pathology; information will stick better this way. Ask questions. There are no stupid questions. Run every decision past a more senior

DOI: 10.1201/9781003350422-14

member of the team initially; the decision-making will get repetitive and simpler with time. You may need to use Google, YouTube, Up-To-Date, DynaMed, or other resources to get quick information. The key here is to be safe and sensible and be aware of your own limitations. Never do anything out of your competence without appropriate supervision.

Not as Glamourous as Advertised

When you imagine life as a CST, you may dream that every day will be spent in theatres, with the entire healthcare team there to help you progress. Unfortunately, the reality is that there are multiple competing interests in the healthcare setting. First and foremost, patient safety and service provision are key outcomes within the NHS. Often, you will feel that your training is less important than these system-wide goals. Navigating your space within the healthcare setting takes grit, creativity, and flexibility. As a CST, you may be in a situation where you are the most junior member of a surgical team, meaning that you will be expected to do ward work. Approach the situation with a growth mindset. Try to find opportunities around you. Are there ward-based practical skills you can learn? Are there difficult conversations with patients you can sit in on, even lead? Can you get to the clinic? Are you able to negotiate with your rota coordinator to have ring-fenced time for operating? In some rotations, your training will be subpar, and in these instances, you must escalate this to your educational supervisor and training programme director. Although the situation may not change in time for you, you can ensure that the educational value of a rotation can be improved for your successors.

Emotional Well-Being

CST will have a profound effect on your emotions. You will be dealing with patients who are undergoing life-changing treatment. You will witness when things go wrong. You will experience death. You will encounter angry patients and relatives. You will experience conflict in the workplace. You might feel out of place, undervalued, or bullied. You may find little value in completing the same administrative tasks you did when you were a foundation doctor. You may find difficulty in getting leave to attend life events. You may get to a stage when you are tired or burnt out.

When you are a CST, you need to take time to focus on yourself and your mental health. Speak to those around you. Build a community of trainees who are going through the same thing and debrief with them. Shared pain is halved pain. If possible, include your significant other, friends, parents, and family so they can support you too. Make time for yourself and your hobbies. When things get too tough, get help. Speak to your educational supervisor or occupational health to get this started.

Financial Well-Being

Financially, CST can also be taxing. Exams cost around £1,000. In addition, you will want to attend other events and courses, some of which are mandatory. You may need to budget for international travel and accommodation expenses. Sometimes you will need to pay to get things published. In addition, this is a time when life events – weddings, children, getting on the property ladder – occur. Suddenly you are a doctor but still feel extremely poor.

You need to work on your financial literacy and keep on top of your budget. Make a list of your income and expenditure every month. Try to save at least a couple of hundred pounds per month and try to build a buffer so that you are not living paycheck-to-paycheck. Make sure that you are claiming back on all the study budget you are entitled to. Research different providers for courses. Some courses (e.g. Train the Trainers) may be offered for free locally, as opposed to with a £500 price tag by a national provider.

Leaving Surgical Training

During CST, some individuals will realise that surgery is not for them. This is all right. Make this decision proudly and use the experiences you have gained during your life as a surgical trainee to become a better version of yourself. You have come this far in your medical career, which means that you are a hardworking, intelligent, ambitious individual; do not let anything or anyone take this self-confidence from you. This is not giving up, it is just choosing a new path. Remember, this is your life and you have to make it what you want.

chapter fourteen

To F3 or Not to F3

Alex Meredith-Hardy, Gargi Pandey, Anokha
Oomman Joseph, and Janso Padickakudi Joseph

Introduction

A foundation year 3 (FY3 or F3) typically describes 12 months out of training for doctors who have completed the foundation programme. As a prospective surgical applicant, you may have already asked yourself the question of whether you want 'to F3 or not to F3'. This is an important, personal decision that only you can make. Candidates who do not receive CST posts will default to the F3 year and may need to make arrangements quickly. Other candidates will make a conscious decision to take an F3 year. In this instance, the central question is how/if a potential F3 year can add value to your life, both personally and professionally. You need to make an honest assessment of your short-term and long-term goals. In this chapter, we present both sides of the argument in a bid to empower you to make the decision that is right for you.

Popularity for an F3 year has boomed, with over 65% of foundation doctors doing an F3 in 2019, compared to only 17% in 2010 ([1]). This once 'alternative' route of not directly entering speciality training has therefore become exceedingly popular. It is also becoming more common for doctors to extend their F3 for further years, colloquially known as F4, F5, F6, and beyond. For this chapter, the term F3 applies to all post-foundation doctors' pre-speciality training.

Proceeding Directly to Speciality Training

Since you are reading this book, you are clearly interested in becoming a surgeon. You may be dipping your toes in the water, or you may already be firmly committed. In either case, proceeding from the foundation programme directly into speciality training may be the right course of action if you are ready for the exciting prospect of being a surgical trainee.

By formally being a core surgical trainee, you become a part of the community of surgery in your hospital, regionally and (inter)nationally. This means your training will be structured, you will be supported by your deanery, and training institutions will have responsibilities towards

DOI: 10.1201/9781003350422-15

your progress. It also means that you will have clinical, academic, and professional responsibilities to fulfil. It firmly puts you on the path to becoming a surgeon in minimal time after graduation; this may become more important further down the line (e.g. when applying for higher surgical training where the requirements become more demanding depending on how long ago you graduated).

It is falsely assumed that proceeding directly into speciality training means you cannot have a work-life balance, cannot travel, or cannot make time for outside interests. With good planning, all these things are possible. If you wish, you can choose to train less than full-time. You can take time to get out-of-programme training, experiences, or research. As a core surgical trainee, you will have the safety of job security. Being a core trainee is also a method of trying out this career path and seeing if it suits you and exploring different surgical specialities. You will be entitled to a study leave budget, holiday, and sick pay.

Reasons to Take an F3 Year

You may have made a conscious decision to take an F3 year. People take this year for many reasons, including travelling, working abroad, preparing for training interviews, gaining further experience in a speciality they may not have had exposure to, or simply taking a break. The decision is usually a combination of personal and professional factors.

Foundation doctors may consider 'push' or 'pull' factors as reasons for taking an F3 [2]. Some of these factors are summarised in the following table.

Negative Factors	Positive Factors
• Stressful/negative experience during foundation training	• Natural break on the 'conveyor belt' of medical training
• Burnout	• Control over time and location
• Lack of speciality exposure	• More flexibility
• Feeling unprepared for speciality training	• Perceived work-life balance
• High competition ratios of the chosen speciality	• Financial incentives
• Failed application	• Increased experience in the chosen speciality
• Lack of control over time/location	• Time to build portfolio
	• Time to pursue other interests/hobbies
	• Travelling
	• Volunteering
	• Life milestones
	• Exploring alternative careers

Flexibility and Work-Life Balance

The opportunity to be fully in control of one's time is attractive. Many doctors have spent year after year at school, sixth form, university, and then foundation training and desire a break from the 'conveyor belt' of medical training. The natural break in training after F2 gives a golden opportunity to take back some control.

Bank or Locum Work

Most F3s continue clinical work in some shape or form. You can either work directly on a staff bank for your trust/hospital to cover rota gaps or empty shifts. Alternatively, you can work through a locum agency. One can choose to take a break from the heavy rota. Some F3s take on a couple of shifts a week to pay the bills and have the rest of the time to enjoy life and pursue other interests, projects, and side hustles. On the opposite end of the spectrum, you can also continue to work (more than) full time, but with the comfort of knowing that you can take time off on your own terms. For many F3s, finding a work-life balance is paramount. The flexibility that bank or locum work offers is a huge draw, especially as fixed rotas can make it difficult to plan life. Everyone seems to have heard a horror story of a core surgical trainee being on-call on their wedding day, despite asking for time off in advance!

Financial Incentives

Bank or locum work means can mean you receive significantly higher pay than a core surgical trainee. At present, a core surgical trainee on an average 40-hour week gets a basic pay of around £19/hour pre-tax. This is before additional rostered hours, night duty, and weekend allowance are factored in. In contrast, the average hourly rate of locums working at the same level is about £44/hour. This is also before national insurance deductions, NHS pension contributions, and student loan repayments. It is obvious that working at the locum rate can be very lucrative. However, it is important to note that there is no sick pay for locum doctors. If you were to take time off work due to sickness, you would have no income during that period.

People have used locum incomes to put together deposits for houses, start property renovation projects, go on round-the-world trips, pay off student debt, start investment portfolios, pay for weddings, and many other things. The possibilities are endless with this 'leg-up' to starting financial independence.

Career Exploration

It is common for foundation doctors to feel uncertain about which speciality training to apply for. It is one of the biggest decisions in your life, and it is reasonable to give yourself the time and space to consider what you want to spend the rest of your professional life doing. Foundation training provides a four-month experience in just six specialities. You may have had little choice in your allocation of rotations. Some niche specialities like ophthalmology do not have foundation trainees, so an F3 year may be a great opportunity to experience this. You may not have rotated through your surgical speciality of choice. During foundation training, you may not have spent much (or any!) time in theatre, despite doing surgical jobs. The F3 year allows you to choose jobs that will give you better exposure to your chosen speciality.

The F3 year is also an opportunity to gain experience in non-clinical roles if this is something that interests you. Examples include medical writing, research, podcasting, YouTubing, management consultancy, health tech, global health policy, and business – the list is endless. You may wish to pursue further education, such as a master's or PhD, an art foundation year, or even a carpentry course. Anything is possible! It is just a matter of deciding how you want to spend your time and planning how you are going to do it.

Portfolio Building

Surgery is a competitive speciality with high applicant-to-post ratios. Although the applicant specifications change every year, there are almost always points for demonstrating teaching commitments, leadership, research, audits, and commitment to the speciality. Although it is possible to build an excellent portfolio during foundation years, you can use the year to really sharpen your portfolio and secure maximum points.

Research and publications are notoriously difficult to get unless you are in the right place at the right time, know the right people, or are genuinely an academic-minded person. The F3 is a brilliant chance to meet people, network, and importantly have the time to get stuck into projects which might lead to presentations and publications, enabling you to finally tick that box.

Locum Agency, Bank Locum, or Clinical/ Teaching Fellowship?

When deciding to take on clinical work in your F3 year, there are several different routes you can go down. You can sign up to the hospital/trust staff bank where you completed your foundation training. The advantage of this is that you will know the institution, the people, the rota coordinators, and the way things work. You will be agile with the IT systems and internal processes, causing the least angst on shifts.

An alternative is to sign up to work for a locum agency. Agents will find work to suit your experience and needs. The benefit of this is that recruitment agents contact you directly with opportunities of which you then have a choice. This route can be the most lucrative. Rates can be negotiated through the locum agent on your behalf. The downsides of locum work are that it can be unpredictable. You must be flexible. You should be ready to pick up last-minute shifts; sometimes at hospitals, you have not worked at before. Some people can find this stressful as you may not always have a predictable source of income. Being in a new hospital without induction or IT training can also be challenging. In general, there is usually work available if you are flexible and prepared to work in different departments and maybe even different hospitals. The other big downside is that you will not qualify for any sick pay.

Clinical and teaching fellowships are another popular option for doctors wanting to continue clinical work during their F3 years. The advantage of these is that they are a great opportunity to gain a solid experience in a chosen speciality. This can be outstanding on a CV and can help with networking. Some of these posts are designed specifically with the F3 doctor in mind. There may be elements in the job description aimed to appeal to those wanting to improve their portfolio, such as allocated time for research, audits, or teaching. Some posts even offer to fund for medical education qualifications. Clinical or teaching fellowships can be competitive to get into but have immense potential for portfolio development. Clinical fellows usually have the same policy for booking annual leave as trainees. They do qualify for pension contributions and sick pay. The downside is that clinical fellows are usually relied on for service provision and are therefore put on the normal F2/SHO rota. This may include on-call, weekends, and nights without the enhanced pay of a locum shift. If you know you want to be a core surgical trainee but were not successful in your application, this may be the option best suited to you.

Working Abroad

Another very popular option for many F3 doctors is to move and work abroad. Many opportunities exist around the world, and medicine is like a passport! You may wish to do volunteer work, combine working with travelling, or seek a permanent relocation. Many UK doctors spend their F3 in Australia, New Zealand, or South Africa. Some never come back!

If you intend to work abroad you need to start this process early, as there will be visa and medical regulatory requirement to fulfil.

Reasons to Proceed to CST	Reasons to Do an F3 Year
Rights and responsibilities of being a core surgical trainee	Flexibility
Structured training	Control over time
Defined expectations	Perceived work-life balance
Deanery support	Potential financial earnings
Sense of identity as a surgeon	Portfolio building
Minimum time after graduation	Freedom for long periods of travel
Ability to try a surgical career	Working abroad
Actively explore surgical specialities	Exploration of interests/careers outside of medicine
Job security	
Predictable rotations	
Rotas in advance	
Study leave, holiday, and sick pay entitlements	

Case Study: Alex Meredith-Hardy

I came across the concept of F3 whilst at medical school when I met an inspiring teaching fellow who spent several incredible years in Australia before coming back to the UK.

Progressing through foundation years, I realised I wanted more time to decide on a speciality, improve my CV, and go travelling. So F3 felt like the right choice to make. I had an incredible year, but due to the consequences of COVID-19, I went on to take an F4 year.

I was keen to gain more teaching experience during my F3 and was lucky enough to secure a part-time job as a teaching fellow and anatomy demonstrator at Barts and the London School of Medicine. This was a fantastic experience as I was able to develop as a teacher, gain a lot more confidence in anatomy, and get involved in several projects with the other fellows which fortunately led to a poster presentation and a publication.

I worked full time with several extended breaks spread throughout the year ranging between one to two weeks to three months. I rarely worked weekends and chose not to do any night shifts. I achieved a good work-life balance and found the freedom to choose when to work extremely liberating as I had more time for things like exercise, seeing friends and family, reading, and painting.

I was also able to do some humanitarian work during the F3 year with Medical Volunteers International (MVI), which runs clinics in the Moria

Refugee Camp in Lesbos, Greece, the biggest refugee camp in Europe. I flew out just before Christmas in the middle of lockdown and had an extremely humbling and fascinating experience working with refugees there. I am so glad that I was able to go. I am looking forward to the prospect of going back as a volunteer with more surgical experience.

As a graduate entry student who had been studying for a long time, I had accrued a lot of student debt with little savings despite working part-time through both degrees. I saw F3 as an opportunity to do locum work and take control of my finances. With the locum work, I took in the F3 year I was able to pay off my overdraft and save for my wedding. I was also able to go on wonderful holidays, replace my 12-year-old laptop, and enjoy living in London!

In my F4 year, I worked in the breast and endocrine unit as a locum senior house officer. The flexibility that my breast surgery job offered me meant that I was able to go on two incredible trips, the first being a trip to the Caribbean and the USA and the second a three-month backpacking trip with my husband around Central America. Highlights of my travels include learning Spanish, staying with a local host family in a village on the shore of Lake Atitlan in Guatemala, volunteering in a biological research station only accessible by boat in the Tortuguero National Park in Costa Rica, spending every day outside in nature, hiking mountains and volcanoes, scuba diving, salsa dancing, seeing amazing wildlife, meeting inspiring people, reading books, and of course, getting to travel and share countless special times with my husband. I found out that I had got a CST training number whilst in a hostel in Guatemala, which was a very memorable day filled with the realisation that my life was all about to change once back in the UK.

Although travelling is arguably not directly career-enhancing, the things that I learned and the experiences that I had were certainly life-enhancing for me. In a way, they made me even more motivated to throw myself fully into CST. Many of my consultants were incredibly supportive of me going away, and some even mentioned regretting not having been able to do these things in their younger lives. So if you enjoy travelling and you are on the fence about taking an F3, then my advice is to take this rare opportunity to get away, completely disconnect from normal life, and have some real adventures before getting stuck into training! The world is your oyster!

Case Study: Gargi Pandey

I completed my foundation year 2 in 2020 when my exposure to different specialities was limited due to the COVID-19 pandemic. I enjoyed my surgical rotation during the foundation programme but did not see myself as a general surgeon. After discussions with friends and colleagues,

I wanted to give ENT a try. ENT is a surgical speciality that also involves medical management, treats all ages, and has a variety of subspecialities.

I managed to organise a taster week during my FY2 year before the pandemic. During this time, I met a female ENT surgeon that inspired me. Everyone I met was so encouraging, and nobody had the stereotypical superior surgical personality. It felt like home. I applied to Core Surgical Training that year on the advice of one of the registrars and was successful in gaining a number in an ENT-themed programme, but I was still keen on taking a year out for three reasons. Firstly, I was not sure if ENT was surgical speciality for me, and I wanted to get more exposure. Secondly, I wanted to do some travelling. Finally, I wanted to do some locum shifts and save for a flat deposit. I was fed up with spending money on rent in London.

Rejecting a training number is a difficult decision. Most of my seniors advised me to take the job as I may not be able to get the number again the following year. However, because of COVID-19, I was also unable to get the surgical experience I needed to decide if ENT was for me. Also, the job I was offered was not my top choice; therefore, I felt I had nothing to lose.

I rejected my offer and instead began my search for the perfect FY3 job. As I did not accept the offer before rejecting it, future applications were not affected. However, if you reject it after accepting the offer, you do have to declare it on your application the following year.

I would advise those wishing to take an F3 year to apply for CST training during FY2 anyway as this will demonstrate any gaps you have in your application and show you what you need to focus on in the coming year to make your application stronger.

Applying during FY2 meant I had my portfolio ready and therefore could concentrate on collecting more points with new projects rather than chasing evidence. I also knew what to expect at the interview stage and exactly how to prepare for the following application year.

I began my search for suitable jobs using the NHS jobs website. I needed to plan a year that was productive but also enjoyable. I narrowed it down to two jobs: anatomy demonstrator or ENT junior clinical fellow. Being an anatomy demonstrator had always been on my list as I heard about all it had to offer. Some anatomy demonstrator jobs offer mentorship for MRCS examinations and the opportunity to study for a fully funded PGCert in medical education. Both elements result in high scoring in the CST self-assessment.

I received an offer for one anatomy demonstrator job and one clinical fellow job. The clinical fellow job would give me exposure to ENT and help me figure out if this was speciality for me. I felt this was important, so I chose the ENT fellow job, and I was extremely satisfied with my decision.

I did the ENT fellow job for six months. This job luckily was not very busy (this is a rarity I must admit). During my time I studied for MRCS Part A and was luckily given study leave for preparation and the exam itself. I highly recommend sitting this exam prior to training, as it takes the pressure off during CST.

My supervisor took me through the self-assessment application and offered ideas on how to gain maximum points in the minimum amount of time. I undertook a teaching programme on the ward. I did a quality improvement project that I presented at a conference in the same year. The hospital also ran a train-the-trainers course before the evidence deadline. So my second original job option covered even more elements of the self-assessment criteria.

I also worked with other SHOs who were also applying. We started interview preparation together and did mock interviews for each other and with registrars. All of this helped to maximise my success in CST applications. I had done so many mock interviews that I was no longer nervous about the real deal. This all led to a much higher ranking in this application period and an ENT themed job in London. After the first six months, I decided to locum for the remainder of the year. I signed up for a locum agency, but instead of doing ad hoc shifts, I signed up for a long-term locum. I found this extremely rewarding as I felt part of a team and had regular income, but still I could request leave whenever I wanted. This added value to my year as I was able to see my family, go to family events and friends' weddings, and also save money for a deposit. This meant I started my CST job in my own flat!

References

1. Silverton R, Freeth D. The F3 phenomenon: Exploring a new norm and its implications. 2018 [cited 2022 Oct 31]. Available from: www.hee.nhs.uk
2. Church HR, Agius SJ. The F3 phenomenon: Early-career training breaks in medical training. A scoping review. Med Educ 2021;55(9):1033–46. Available from: https://pubmed.ncbi.nlm.nih.gov/33945168/

chapter fifteen

Medical Students – Planning a Career in Surgery

Rose Kurian Thomas

Introduction

Surgical training is a notably competitive and challenging medical discipline to gain entry into.[1] Therefore, it is crucial to be meticulous and well-prepared when you apply. Typically, having graduated from medical school, you have two to three years of experience working as a foundation doctor before making competitive applications for surgical training posts. The key to a successful application is a well-developed surgical portfolio. Whilst it is feasible to achieve the necessary requirements for an eminent application during the two/three years as a junior doctor, the medical school offers the luxury of five or six years of time to prepare for this. Medical students have substantially more free time and flexibility (without the stressors of working life) to plan and seek out early opportunities to fulfil the requirements of a strong surgical candidate.

This chapter will outline ways you can maximise your opportunities as a medical student to widen your horizons. It will show you how to strengthen your application with adequate surgical experience and simplify the surgical application process – if you decided to go down this route. Even if you are undetermined about surgery, this chapter will facilitate prospects to explore your surgical interests during medical school.

Joining Surgical Societies

Surgical societies are student-led organisations within medical schools to widen medical students' awareness and aspirations in surgery. These societies coordinate a range of opportunities, including surgical skills workshops, career talks, surgical work experience arrangements, mentorship schemes, and conferences. Career guiding opportunities and expedited readiness for a career in surgery are two of the most noted benefits of surgical society membership for medical students.[2] Furthermore, medical students predominantly rely on surgical career

DOI: 10.1201/9781003350422-16

guidance from their mentors.[3] Comprehensive involvement in your medical school's surgical society does the groundwork for you to network with established surgeons, identify your mentors, and shape your career decisions.

Most medical schools in the UK should have an established surgical society. If, however, this is not the case for your medical school, then this is a key opportunity for you to demonstrate your dedication to the speciality. Likewise, holding positions of responsibility within the surgical society, implementing positive changes, setting up society activities, or creating subspecialised groups can all show commitment to the field of surgery. Such positions are also fundamental to hone your interpersonal skills, such as leadership, communication, and teamwork.

Conferences

Surgical organisations annually organise conferences where like-minded individuals and experts congregate to share knowledge, interests, and up-to-date advances in surgery. These can be regional, national, or international conferences. Attending surgical conferences is not mandatory, but there are numerous substantial benefits for medical students which cannot be substituted in lecture theatres or hospital settings.[4]

Conferences offer the valuable opportunity to submit abstracts to present surgically relevant projects you have undertaken. This can be quality improvement projects, research findings, or audits. Successful abstract submission is an outlet for a poster or an oral presentation about your project, and some conferences offer prizes for scoring highly in your abstract, poster, or oral presentations. These achievements hold substantial weight in future applications for surgical training.

A conference offers a common language for medical students to connect with other participants and experts attending the conference. Ask all the questions you have with no hesitation; the prefix 'I am a medical student' also offers a free ticket for your curiosity, no matter how advanced or elementary the question is. Your eagerness is highly acknowledged, and most surgeons are ardent supporters of conveying their vast knowledge to interested students. Such interactions are great for developing connections with adept surgeons, and these contacts can be maintained through a simple email to express your appreciation for meeting them. This is also a way of signposting further correspondences regarding questions, advice, and opportunities in surgery.

Your first national or international conference can be nerve-wracking, and amidst formal networking with specialists, you may feel out of depth. One of the best ways to ease into attending conferences is to familiarise yourself with student-led conferences at your medical school and other medical schools. These conferences are designed exclusively for medical students on topical matters pertinent to students. They can provide a better understanding of conferences and improve your confidence in both presenting your work and networking with renowned surgeons.

Courses

Whilst the medical school curriculum is great for theoretical knowledge, the opportunities for hands-on practice of surgical skills can often be limited and varies based on medical school.[5] Courses on practising surgical skills, using laparoscopic equipment, and surgical simulation sessions are very useful additions to the undergraduate curriculum. They improve confidence in basic skills learnt at medical school, allow you to upskill in advanced surgical skills, and explore interests beyond the curriculum.[6], [7] The best part is most conference workshops and surgical courses offer these remarkable opportunities at heavily discounted prices for students!

The student affiliate network at the Royal College of Surgeons of Edinburgh is aimed at augmenting medical students' practical experiences of surgery. The Royal College of Surgeons of England also offers affiliate membership. Annual membership for both is around £5–15 for medical students and entitles access to an abundant source of opportunities, including subsidised surgical courses and educational webinars. These opportunities refine your skillsets, consolidate your portfolio, and give you valuable continuing professional development points early on in your career.

In the following table are some of the courses offered by the affiliate network and other providers. It also includes their estimated costs and length of the course.

Surgical Course	Provider	Cost	Length
Foundations of Clinical Surgery[8]	Royal College of Surgeons of Edinburgh	£120–135	2 days
Future Surgeons: Key Skills[8]	Royal College of Surgeons of Edinburgh	£110	1 day
Plastering Techniques for Fracture Treatment[8]	Royal College of Surgeons of Edinburgh	£124–138	1 day

(continued)

(Continued)

Surgical Course	Provider	Cost	Length
RCSEd Cadaveric Intermediate Open Abdominal Surgery Course[8]	Royal College of Surgeons of Edinburgh	£45–75	2 days
Foundations of Gastrointestinal Surgery[8]	Royal College of Surgeons of Edinburgh	£120–135	2 days
Surgical Anatomy of the Head and Neck: A Study Day[8] Surgical Anatomy of the Trunk: A Study Day[8] Surgical Anatomy of the Limbs: A Study Day[8]	Royal College of Surgeons of Edinburgh	£85 each	Each 1 day
Surgical Skills for Students and Health Professionals[9]	Royal College of Surgeons of England	£99	1 day
Systematic Training in Acute Illness Recognition and Treatment (START)[10]	Royal College of Surgeons of England	£139	1 day
Foundation skills in Surgery[11]	Royal College of Physicians and Surgeons of Glasgow	£85–120	1 day
Basic Orthopaedic Procedural Skills[12]	Royal College of Physicians and Surgeons of Glasgow	£149–189	1 day

Competitions and Grants

There are plenty of competitions and grants available to medical students for various subspecialities of surgery. Many medical students are not aware of these opportunities. Making time for these accomplishments as an overstretched junior doctor is challenging and demanding; however, as a medical student, you have the knowledge base and timeframe for partaking in these opportunities. In addition, surgically relevant prizes and grants from competitions hold significant value in terms of portfolio points in your future surgical applications. Therefore, save your future doctor self from added work and pressure by exploring these opportunities early during medical school!

Here is a list of some relevant surgical organisations and the annual competitions and grants they offer. This is not an exhaustive list:

Organisation	Description
Royal Society of Medicine[13]	Offers a plethora of medical student prizes in various specialities including surgical specialities. Prize competitions include the following: 1. Essay prizes 2. Elective awards 3. Poster and presentation prizes 4. Bursaries and travelling fellowships
British Society for Dermatological Surgery[14]	Medical student essay prizes
British Orthopaedic Association[15]	
British Association of Urological Surgeons[16]	
Student and Foundation Doctors in Otolaryngology (SFO-UK)[17]	• SFO Undergraduate Essay Prize • SFO UK Innovative Education Prize • SFO UK Elective Prize
Royal College of Surgeons of Edinburgh[18]	RCSEd and Vascutek cardiothoracic surgery placements: Opportunity to undertake placements in cardiothoracic surgery at renowned cardiothoracic centres in the UK
Royal College of Surgeons of England[19]	Professor Harold Ellis Medical Student Prize for Surgery – Abstract Submission
Royal College of Surgeons of Edinburgh[20]	Lister Surgical Skills National Competition
Royal College of Surgeons of Ireland[21]	National Surgical Skills Competition
Royal College of Surgeons of Edinburgh[22]	RCSEd and Medtronic Surgical Skills Competition
Royal College of Surgeons of England[23]	Grants for medical students who are interested doing an intercalated Bachelor of Science degree related to surgery
Royal College of Surgeons of Ireland[24]	Barker Dissection Award – for the student achieving highest grade for dissection and written report
Royal College of Surgeons of Ireland[24]	Sayed-Hanson Memorial Award – for the student achieving highest grade for head, neck, and neuroanatomy

Electives

An elective is a self-organised placement that is usually completed as part of the final year of medical school. This can be done within the UK or internationally. It is one of the most enthralling and memorable chapters of medical school and can be done alone or with friends.

Undertaking a surgically relevant elective is a comprehensive way of expanding your curiosity in surgery. This is also a recognised accomplishment in your future surgical training applications as it demonstrates dedication to surgery. Surgical electives can entail a variety of experiences, including and not limited to clinical experience, research, surgical medical technology, and surgical medical education.

So far in this chapter, we have discussed the significance of having a surgical mentor and expanding your surgical network of contacts. Applying for electives is a fine example of how these contacts can be invaluable to organising a fruitful and rewarding experience. Be prepared to send out lots of emails!

When pondering whether to stay in the UK or go internationally, let us have a look at the pros and cons of each:

The main advantage of an international elective is the opportunity to build a global network of professional contacts who can inspire and improve your practical skills and knowledge in surgical practices not commonly seen in the UK. The ability to travel and immerse in all that a foreign country has to offer provides the chance to develop cultural competence – an important ability to foster in the NHS, given the huge cultural diversity of patients we have.

However, international electives are significantly more expensive and require meticulous planning with more paperwork completion. This is primarily because there is a more scrupulous approval process due to the increased health and safety risks associated with an international elective – although the type of risk is dependent on which country you go to.

The disadvantages of an international elective are the advantages of a UK elective – they are comparatively easier to coordinate with fewer paperwork and less associated costs. UK electives are great ways of expanding your surgical network within the UK as the UK is the centre of internationally renowned surgical institutions and hospitals with highly acknowledged surgeons. It is important to note that previous surgical experiences at UK medical schools could already provide you with what a clinical surgical elective in the UK has to offer. Therefore, surgical research opportunities or clinical placements in major UK specialist surgical centres are good alternatives to broaden your horizons in surgery and to see and do what you may not have already seen/done at medical school.

Now if you decide on an international elective, a dichotomy between an elective in a developing country and a developed country exists. An elective in a developing country can provide better exposure to global health issues and awareness of prevailing health inequalities around the world. This also facilitates more opportunities to be involved in sustainable health improvement projects for local communities. In addition, the vast variety of conditions in developing nations and the differences in surgical practices compared to the developed world can widen your awareness of conditions and surgical techniques that are not common in the UK. You may also have more hands-on experience and opportunities to practice procedures. However, this goes hand in hand with feeling thrown into the deep end in quite an unfamiliar healthcare system because you could be assumed to take on roles beyond your limitations or unsupervised due to limited resources and/or understaffed circumstances.[25]

Whilst there is a curtailed variety of conditions to experience in developed countries than developing countries, you are more likely to feel comfortable doing a surgical elective in a developed country as it is likely to have a similar supported and supervised healthcare environment to the UK. Developed countries also offer the opportunity to work in highly reputable institutions using state-of-the-art technology which can improve your awareness of advanced surgical practices and novel technology. There is also more scope for being involved in research projects funded by these institutions.

An extensive range of organisations offers student grants for surgically relevant electives. It is useful to be aware of them so you can apply before the deadlines pass. Here are some to consider:

Organisation	Description
The Beit Trust[26]	Bursaries for electives in Zimbabwe, Malawi, and Zambia – £700–1,000
The British Association of Plastic Reconstructive and Aesthetic Surgeons[26]	Support for partaking in research, travel, and elective related to plastic surgery – £500
Edward Boyle Elective Bursary[26]	Support for elective comprising in low-/middle-income countries within the Commonwealth – £500
Medical Women's Federation[26]	Grants to support female students in their electives – £100–500
Royal College of Surgeons of Edinburgh[27]	• Russel Trust Bursary for surgical elective abroad • Bursaries for undergraduate elective or vacation studies • Cardiothoracic surgery elective travel awards • RCSEd/Blinks trust elective travel awards – £250 • Bursaries for elective placements in Africa

(continued)

(Continued)

Organisation	Description
Royal College of Surgeons of England[28]	• RCS England Elective Prize in Surgery for surgical elective in developing country – £500 • PKK and SK elective fellowships to undertake an elective in surgery in India – £1,000
Royal College of Physicians and Surgeons of Glasgow[29]	Medical elective scholarship – maximum of £1,000
The Simmonds Bursary[26]	Financial support for undertaking elective in UK or internationally *with* research – £250

Case Study: Rose Kurian Thomas

My initial exposure to surgery began in my first year of medical school. I joined as a subcommittee member of my medical school's surgical society. There are numerous advantages to this as it requires no prior experience, you can gain full insight into society, and it paves the way to holding more senior positions. As a committee member, I had exclusive free access to all events hosted by the society including surgical webinars, skills development workshops, career talks, and surgical symposiums.

COVID-19 disrupted my surgical placement, so I did not actually get into an operating theatre until my fifth year of medical school. But early involvement in the aforementioned external opportunities gave me insight into different surgical specialities and built my foundation in pertinent surgical practices, such as suturing, abscess drainage, and surgical drain insertions.

Finally, when I did get into operating theatres, I was truly mind-blown by the surgeons and surgeries I observed, including on-pump coronary artery bypass and renal transplant surgeries. I feel very lucky to have worked with highly established surgeons who were keen to reciprocate my interest and develop my practical skills. I was taught different surgical knot-tying techniques, allowed to close up on patients, trained to handle the laparoscopic equipment, and given countless opportunities to scrub and assist in surgeries. I enjoyed this placement so much that this was probably the only placement at medical school I stayed longer than 12 hours in one day! A poignant memory I have is of a procedure that had a major artery suddenly bleed – like a jet spray. The surgeons and other team members were poised, fast-acting in all their decisions, and swift to retrieve the patient to haemodynamic stability. Observing this in action was a terrifying but enlightening experience – one of my most inspiring observations.

I have been very fortunate to cultivate good relationships with surgeons I have met in my journey of medicine thus far. Two of them have guided me from the very beginning when I was an inexperienced school student interested in medicine to now as a final year medical student. I consider them my medical parents, truly insightful senior surgeons whom I go to for my career and life queries. One such example was discussing which degree to intercalate in for my BSc. I ended up doing a BSc in medical sciences with management because of the following reasons:

1. The modules interested me.
2. It is unrelated to clinical medicine. Imperial was one of the only two universities at the time offering intercalation in management.
3. This will give me an extra range of unique skills and knowledge that can set me apart.

Moreover, they have also shown me the realities of life as a surgeon and kept me grounded, focused, and motivated in my career. I am grateful for their outpouring of wisdom and the opportunities they have offered me. Writing this chapter for this book is an example of one of the opportunities that they have opened up for me as mentors.

During one of my placements, I came across my next mentor. Her practice of medicine and interpersonal qualities inspired me to what sort of doctor I wanted to become. I took on a project with her, which we presented at the Royal College of Obstetricians and Gynaecologists World Congress. This was a very rewarding opportunity for me because our abstract was one of the highest-scoring abstracts and was published in the *British Journal of Obstetrics and Gynaecology*.

My other mentor is more junior in his surgical training. We have more of an easygoing and open relationship, which created a safe space to make many mistakes with no expectations or judgement! I got plenty of learning done and received valuable individualised feedback! He gave me insight into the significance of having signed written evidence of all the activities I partake in, such as courses, projects, teaching experiences, and involvement in societies. I also realised having a logbook and creating a habit of recording procedures/surgeries is very important for applications because the number of personally involved cases is vital for your portfolio.

Now that I come to the end of my medical school life, I am really excited about my elective (and of course to never sit medical school exams again). I was always certain I wanted an international elective because I was fortunate to have adequate exposure already in the UK, and since I am a UK citizen, the NHS bursary covers part of my accommodation costs for the elective country. The real question was, should I go to a developing or developed country? I already had the experience of undertaking a medical project in Uganda and therefore have obtained the desired exposure of medical practice in the developing world. So to broaden my horizons, I decided to go to a developed country, such as Canada or Australia, because I am interested in working in these countries in the future. After sending many emails, I finally got accepted for an elective in renal transplant surgery at Royal Adelaide Hospital, Australia, my last official placement as a medical student.

So that is me ending one big chapter (both figuratively and literally) – looking forward to seeing where life takes me!

References

1. Health Education England. (2021) *2021 Competition Ratios Nationally Advertised Vacancies.* Available at: https://specialtytraining.hee.nhs.uk/Portals/1/2021%20 Competition%20Ratios_1.pdf (Accessed: November 20, 2022).
2. Ologunde, R., Rufai, S.R. and Lee, A.H.Y. (2015) "Inspiring Tomorrow's Surgeons: The Benefits of Student Surgical Society Membership☆?>," *Journal of Surgical Education*, 72(1), pp. 104–107. Available at: https://doi.org/10.1016/j. jsurg.2014.06.004.
3. Sutton, P.A. et al. (2014) "Attitudes, Motivators, and Barriers to a Career in Surgery: A National Study of UK Undergraduate Medical Students," *Journal of Surgical Education*, 71(5), pp. 662–667. Available at: https://doi.org/10.1016/j. jsurg.2014.03.005.
4. Mishra, S. (2016) "Do Medical Conferences Have a Role to Play? Sharpen the Saw," *Indian Heart Journal*, 68(2), pp. 111–113. Available at: https://doi. org/10.1016/j.ihj.2016.03.011.
5. Hakim, M. et al. (2019) "Surgical Skills Workshops Should Be a Part of the United Kingdom Undergraduate Medical Curriculum," *Cureus* [Preprint]. Available at: https://doi.org/10.7759/cureus.4642.
6. Seo, H.S. et al. (2017) "A One-Day Surgical-Skill Training Course for Medical Students' Improved Surgical Skills and Increased Interest in Surgery as a Career," *BMC Medical Education*, 17(1). Available at: https://doi.org/10.1186/ s12909-017-1106-x.
7. Kuo, L. et al. (2022) "Impact of an In-Person Small Group Surgical Skills Course for Preclinical Medical Students in an Era of Increased e-Learning," *Surgery Open Science*, 10, pp. 148–155. Available at: https://doi.org/10.1016/j. sopen.2022.09.004.
8. Royal College of Surgeons of Edinburgh. (no date) *Courses, Events & Exams: Rcsed, The Royal College of Surgeons of Edinburgh*. Available at: www.rcsed. ac.uk/courses-events-exams-search-results-page?SearchType=Course (Accessed: November 25, 2022).
9. *Surgical Skills for Students and Health Professionals*. Royal College of Surgeons of England. Available at: www.rcseng.ac.uk/education-and-exams/courses/ search/surgical-skills-for-students-and-health-professionals/ (Accessed: December 22, 2022).
10. *Systematic Training in Acute Illness Recognition and Treatment START.* Royal College of Surgeons of England. Available at: www.rcseng.ac.uk/

education-and-exams/courses/search/systematic-training-in-acute-illness-recognition-and-treatment-start/ (Accessed: December 22, 2022).

11. *Foundation Skills in Surgery*. Royal College of Physicians and Surgeons of Glasgow. Available at: https://community.rcpsg.ac.uk/event/view/foundation-skills-in-surgery-25-mar-23 (Accessed: December 24, 2022).

12. *Basic Orthopedic Procedural Skills*. Royal College of Physicians and Surgeons of Glasgow. Available at: https://community.rcpsg.ac.uk/event/view/basic-orthopaedic-procedural-skills-28-feb-23 (Accessed: December 24, 2022).

13. Royal Society of Medicine. (2022) *Prizes for Students, the Royal Society of Medicine.* Available at: www.rsm.ac.uk/prizes-and-awards/prizes-for-students/ (Accessed: November 26, 2022).

14. British Society for Dermatological Society. (2022) *Medical Student Essay Prize, British Society for Dermatological Surgery.* Available at: https://bsds.org.uk/awards/medical-student-essay-prize/ (Accessed: November 26, 2022).

15. Boa, B.O.A. (2022) *Medical Student Essay Prize, British Orthopaedic Association.* Available at: www.boa.ac.uk/learning-and-events/fellowships-awards/awards-and-prizes/medical-student-essay-prize.html (Accessed: November 26, 2022).

16. *Essay Competition.* (2022) *The British Association of Urological Surgeons.* Available at: www.baus.org.uk/professionals/sections/essay_competition.aspx (Accessed: November 26, 2022).

17. *Prizes and Awards.* (2022) *ENT UK.* Available at: www.entuk.org/about/groups/SFO/prizes_and_awards.aspx (Accessed: November 26, 2022).

18. The Royal College of Surgeons of Edinburgh. (2022) *Hospital Placement Opportunities for Undergraduates, the Royal College of Surgeons of Edinburgh.* Available at: www.rcsed.ac.uk/professional-support-development-resources/career-support/career-advice-for-medical-students/hospital-placement-opportunities-for-undergraduates (Accessed: November 26, 2022).

19. *Medical Student Prizes.* Royal College of Surgeons of England. Available at: www.rcseng.ac.uk/careers-in-surgery/medical-students/prizes-for-medical-students/ (Accessed: December 24, 2022).

20. *Medical Student Prizes.* The Association of Surgeons in Training. Available at: www.asit.org/resources/medical-students/prizes/res1192 (Accessed: December 24, 2022).

21. *RCSI Hosts National Surgical Skills Competition 2020.* Royal College of Surgeons of Ireland. Available at: www.rcsi.com/dublin/news-and-events/news/news-article/2020/02/rcsi-hosts-national-surgical-skills-competition-2020 (Accessed: December 24, 2022).

22. *Competition Details: RCSEd and Medtronic Surgical Skills Competition 2022.* The Royal College of Surgeons of Edinburgh. Available at: www.rcsed.ac.uk/events-courses/competition-details-rcsed-and-medtronic-surgical-skills-competition-2022 (Accessed: December 24, 2022).

23. *Awards and Grants.* Royal College of Surgeons of England. Available at: www.rcseng.ac.uk/standards-and-research/research/fellowships-awards-grants/awards-and-grants/ (Accessed: December 24, 2022).

24. *Student Academic Awards Offered by the School of Medicine.* Royal College of Surgeons of Ireland. Available at: www.rcsi.com/dublin/student-life/student-opportunities/student-academic-awards/school-of-medicine (Accessed: December 24, 2022).

25. Tahiri, Y. (2020) "Impressions on an Elective Abroad," *McGill Journal of Medicine*, 11(1). Available at: https://doi.org/10.26443/mjm.v11i1.414.
26. Medical Schools Council. (2022) *Elective Bursaries, Medical Schools Council.* Available at: www.medschools.ac.uk/studying-medicine/current-medical-students/elective-bursaries (Accessed: November 29, 2022).
27. Royal College of Surgeons of Edinburgh. (no date) *Student Bursaries: RCSEd, The Royal College of Surgeons of Edinburgh.* Available at: www.rcsed.ac.uk/professional-support-development-resources/grants-jobs-and-placements/research-travel-and-award-opportunities/student-bursaries (Accessed: November 29, 2022).
28. *RCS England Elective Prize in Surgery and the PKK & SK Elective Fellowships.* Royal College of Surgeons of England. Available at: www.rcseng.ac.uk/standards-and-research/research/fellowships-awards-grants/awards-and-grants/medical-student-awards/rcs-elective-prize-in-surgery/ (Accessed: December 24, 2022).
29. *Medical Elective Scholarship.* The Royal College of Physicians and Surgeons of Glasgow. Available at: https://rcpsg.ac.uk/awards-and-scholarships/medical-elective-scholarship#:~:text=We%20offer%20eight%20scholarships%20of,within%20the%20medical%20school%20curriculum (Accessed: December 24, 2022).

chapter sixteen

Women in Surgery

Sharlini Sathananthan and Anokha Oomman Joseph

Introduction

Over the years, even though the number of female medical students has increased, the number of women in surgery is still significantly low. As the global agenda towards gender equality progresses, there is an increasing need for us to acknowledge the matter of gender inequality in the surgical workplace. Surgery continues to be male-dominated, with consultant female surgeons representing only 13.2% of the consultant body in England in 2020 (1).

As surgical registrars who have trained and worked in this field for many years, although the joy from this work has been unparalleled, the unspoken reality of gender bias within the speciality – both conscious and unconscious – has been a sobering experience for us.

Surgery is notorious for traditionally being a male-dominated profession, and as a result, the speciality leads itself to be deeply entrenched structural barriers that can inadvertently impede the career advancement of its female trainees. Although the landscape is rapidly evolving, and we must not take away from the excellent progress that has been made, there is still a lot of work to be done.

Barriers and challenges to a career in surgery for women include gender bias, perceptions of a surgeon, work-life balance, motherhood, and rigid career structures (2). There is a belief held by many that a career in surgery is not compatible with having a healthy work-life balance, a happy marriage or raising children (3).

In this chapter, we will shed light on some of the gender barriers that threaten the progression of so many outstanding women in surgery and impart some advice on how to tackle these issues.

Gender Bias

Many female surgeons experience gender bias in the workplace that can have a negative impact on their performance during training (4) and their overall professional trajectory (5). Up to 66.7% of women in surgery still

DOI: 10.1201/9781003350422-17

experience various forms of discrimination within the workplace and concerningly high dropout rates are reported among female surgeons (6).

Some of these barriers manifest more overtly; others tend to be more subtle microaggressions that gradually erode the confidence that female surgeons have in themselves while at work. Women often cite these barriers as preventing them from evolving into content, happy, independent surgeons with a feeling of control over their careers and simultaneously whole and fulfilling personal lives.

One cannot deny the valuable attributes offered by women in the surgical workplace. Studies report more compassionate and effective leadership, better physician-patient communication, provision of more patient-centric care, and even fewer complication rates in surgeries performed by female surgeons when compared to their counterparts (7). However, for decades now, women have been adapting their lives to male-centric surgical training programmes that were developed with no consideration for the complex needs of women within the speciality.

If you speak to an aspiring female surgeon, she will often tell you that even as a medical student, she was actively discouraged from pursuing a surgical career path by well-intentioned senior doctors and mentors, usually male. Reasons cited would classically include the perceived difficulty of the 'gentle' feminine personality to navigate an uncompromisingly intense, male-dominated workplace and biased accounts of how a surgical career is not compatible with healthy family life for women (8). These presumptions about the unsuitability of a surgical career for women are often ill-informed and have deterred many young women from seriously considering the speciality when there is a possibility that surgery might in fact be a very fulfilling career choice for them.

The perception of female surgeons is an additional problem. Women are often perceived as being weaker, less competent, and less trustworthy than their counterparts. Men are seen as being more suited to the demanding surgical workload. Women in surgery report being judged far more harshly than their male colleagues, leaving them feeling the pressure to reach a much higher standard to prove their worth. Studies show that women who have more familial duties are often treated as being less committed to work by seniors. Perception even in the most literal sense has been highlighted by female surgeons and trainees who felt they were judged by their appearance rather than their capabilities and qualities, resulting in pressure to be extra conscious about their dressing and upkeep (9).

The Stereotypical Surgeon

Subtler grievances include the philosophy perpetuated by many within the speciality that you must have an 'alpha' personality to be a surgeon.

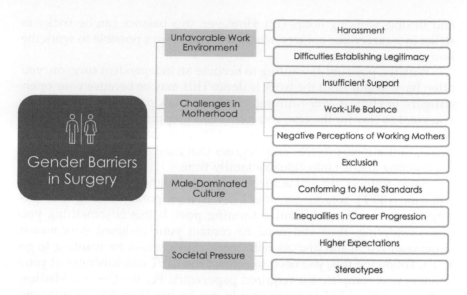

Figure 16.1 Gender barriers faced by women.

Although this is in part due to the high pressures of the strained health-care services that we work in, the idea that women must be exceptionally resilient and tough to work in the profession is an exclusive and damaging one. Sadly, it is often perpetuated by female surgeons themselves, whose own tough workplace personalities have evolved as a by-product of the culture they were trained in. By implicitly making this a prerequisite for being considered a good female surgeon, we run the risk of contributing to a further lack of compassion and empathy within the speciality which it so desperately needs. All that should be required to be a good surgical trainee is a conscientious, safe, and dedicated approach to your work, paired with a progression in competence and the ability to take constructive feedback from your seniors. The idea that certain personalities, genders, and races are more conducive to a career in surgery is inaccurate, and we must be careful that these ideas are not weaponised as forerunners for people's personal prejudices (10).

Work-Life Balance

Surgical training is long and often happens at a time when many women would like to settle down in their personal lives, get married, and have children. Medical students have been deterred from choosing surgery as a speciality because they feel they will not have the balance in life that they want (11). It is good to see the culture around work-life balance evolving with both male and female doctors wanting more time for social activities and flexible working hours (12). However, this balance can be tricky to strike in a career like surgery where it is not always possible to work the hours you are contracted.

With the pressure of wanting to become an independent surgeon, you often have to stay until the work is done. This may be because your operating list or clinic is over-running, you have a sick patient on the ward, or you want to stay for the case you have been prepping all day. The unpredictability of the job means it is often difficult to plan things ahead. The extra publications, projects, and degrees that most surgeons take on during training also eat into valuable family time.

Some trainees try and achieve work-life balance by going less than full-time (LTFT). You can consider LTFT in a temporary or long-term setting if you are in a substantive training post. If this is something you are considering, then you need to contact your assigned educational supervisor (AES) and discuss with them your reasons for wanting to go LTFT. Following this, you need to contact the LTFT administrator at your deanery and complete the required paperwork. Per the General Medical Council (GMC), LTFT training should not be less than 50% of full-time training. In exceptional circumstances, postgraduate deans have the flexibility to reduce this to 20% of full-time training for a maximum of 12 months. It is important that you plan things in advance so that adequate cover can be sorted locally ([13]). Ultimately, the decision you make should be based on what works for you and your situation.

Planning Motherhood and Fertility

Another major barrier that women face when considering a career in surgery is the idea that choosing a career in surgery means that they are rejecting a family life and their chance to have children.

Certainly, some of these concerns have been raised in the literature. Female surgeons are more likely to delay having children compared to male surgeons (14). Some reasons for the delay in having children include long and busy work schedules, not wanting to prolong training, childcare issues, and worries about 'burdening' colleagues (15). Many female surgeons often feel they must pick their career over starting a family.

The average age at first pregnancy is significantly higher in female surgeons because of worries about finishing training and wanting to avoid the negative attitudes of peers and superiors (5). Advanced maternal age then in itself becomes a risk factor for pregnancy-related complications as well as negative fetal and neonatal outcomes.

When female surgeons are finally ready to start a family after they have completed training, a significant number have issues with fertility. A study done in America of female surgeons showed that 32% of the surgeons surveyed reported fertility-related issues, and 84% had under-gone tests for infertility. Out of all the babies born to the surgeons in the study, 13% were conceived using assisted reproductive techniques (16).

The rate of miscarriage is higher in female surgeons compared to female non-surgeons (17). The rate of miscarriage in female surgeons in literature is reported to be between 14.9% (17) and 42% (14). It has also been reported that female surgeons were more likely to experience pregnancy-related complications compared to other non-surgical col-leagues. This may be due to direct reasons, such as long hours of work-ing, prolonged standing, and exposure to surgical smoke, radiation, and anaesthetic gases (5).

Many female surgeons feel that the nature of their work has had a harmful impact on their pregnancy. A Canadian study reported that 31% of the female surgeons surveyed felt their work had adversely affected their pregnancy. This included outcomes such as miscarriage, pre-term labour, hypertension, and pre-eclampsia.

There is no correct time to start a family. Trainees have children in all stages of training, and it really depends on your personal situation. A study in America suggested that female surgeons in training should have fertility-focused educational interventions. This will provide female surgeons with the information required to decide if they want to pur-sue egg preservation and think ahead in terms of family planning, thus allowing them not to miss out on having children later in life (18).

If you are pregnant and in training, continuing surgical training whilst being pregnant can be challenging because of the physical demands of the job whilst experiencing pregnancy-associated symptoms. You can go on maternity leave from 27 weeks and return to work a year later. But most trainees like to take maternity leave close to the delivery date so that the maternity leave clock starts at that point, and they get to spend more time with the baby. It is important that you involve your GP and local occupa-tional health department if you are struggling during the pregnancy, as they can suggest amendments to your work schedule which your depart-ment has to honour.

Leadership and Mentorship

There is a dearth of female surgeons in positions of leadership and senior academic rankings, which results in fewer mentors and role models for women. The Kennedy report has highlighted some of these issues and made recommendations to address these (19).

The purpose of a mentor is to help you plan and navigate your career. Their experience in the field means they are well-placed to guide you in developing your CV, improve your networking abilities, and guide you to appropriate courses that will help you build the skills you need for career advancement (20). You may come across a senior at a workplace you trust and respect and build a relationship with them in which they organically become your mentor. The other way to find a mentor that is separate from your clinical environment is through organisations such as the Association of Surgeons in Training (ASiT) that have a mentorship programme (21) and Women in Surgery (WiS) (1). Mentorship allows trainees to develop leadership and interpersonal skills and achieve their maximum potential.

Tackling the Culture in Surgery

Female surgeons also report dysregulation from the spectrum of misogynistic attitudes and behaviours attributable to the 'boys club culture' within surgery (22). At the far end of this spectrum are the harrowing accounts of sexual abuse and harassment that so many have bravely come forward publicly within the last couple of years (23). Although it has been described as shocking, the reality is many have been aware of this widespread problem for years without the tools to address or improve it. We must appreciate the gravity of this problem, which presents the greatest of threats not just to the basic human right of an individual to feel safe at work but also to the performance and mental well-being of surgeons who are subject to these kinds of abuse.

A problem that goes hand in hand with this is the difficulty in escalating concerns about colleagues and seniors. Due to notoriously nepotistic surgical work environments, there is insufficient support for women who do decide to take workplace concerns further. There are documented limitations in the disciplinary action that can be taken against senior surgeons with only very few cases of reported incidents of sexual abuse or harassment within the speciality resulting in a disciplinary trial. Department-level attempts to conceal and cover up allegations rather than addressing problems in a transparent way are widely reported. Furthermore, there is almost inevitable damage to the career of the perceived 'whistle-blower' who is seen as disrupting the 'status quo' in the process of escalating a concern against a usually very well-established and well-connected senior surgeon (23).

Many working within the speciality will tell you there is an implicit expectation to keep your head down, get on with the work, and have the self-awareness to know that escalating inappropriate behaviour has a high chance of damaging your career prospects. Many who have left the career will tell you the way a complaint was handled was the final straw. If we are to make the speciality somewhere that women want to work, this must change.

What Needs to Change?

The challenges faced by women in surgery, especially the conflict between familial responsibilities and surgical duties, often lead to women feeling like they are always sacrificing one for another in a way that is detrimental to their self-esteem. The guilt from this can deter female surgeons from continuing in their chosen career path. Studies have shown that this is the biggest reason for the low uptake of a career in surgery and for drop-out from a surgical career in women (6, 8, 22). It is time to realise that we are asking women to pay too great a price to establish successful careers in this discipline, and more must be done to make surgery a more holistically supportive and attractive speciality to its female members.

So how do we help address the problem? And how can *you* be success-ful, instil confidence in yourself, and drive change at the very start of your journey as a young aspiring surgeon?

Recommendations

Firstly, although it is important to be aware of the guidance and opinions of those in positions of seniority, you must develop the ability to criti-cally appraise and challenge this information. One of the most impor-tant lessons to be learned as a surgical trainee is the benefit of accepting feedback and counsel from those around you. This has undoubtedly played a significant role in our growth. It is often much more difficult for us to see where we need to improve like our peers and seniors can. However, you must develop the tools to dissect and evaluate what is appropriate and constructive and what is irrelevant. Tact and gracious-ness go a long way in managing conversations with those who are not imparting knowledge that is useful to you, especially when that advice is well-intentioned.

Secondly, you should proactively engage with positive, inspirational role models who do exist within the speciality. Women in Surgery (WiS) is a national initiative that provides support to women pursuing a surgical career. It aims to empower female surgeons through mentorship, network-ing, and education (1). It gives visibility to inspirational female surgeons who are navigating successful professional and personal lives and sheds light on their stories. Furthermore, the organisation is constantly challeng-ing the barriers that threaten the progress of women within surgery and never fails to celebrate examples of excellent trainers, trainees, and men-tors within the profession. Interacting with a role model to whom you can relate is all it takes to give you the drive to succeed.

Seeking out a variety of relatable, motivating, and supportive men-tors is perhaps one of the most helpful things you can do to help yourself through difficult periods in your journey as a surgeon. There are also a variety of other support groups available. We would like to pay special homage to two Facebook groups for doctors; the first is called 'Tea & Empathy', which is an informal, peer-to-peer support network that provides a platform for anonymous advice on a whole range of issues that affect healthcare professionals. The second is called 'Physician mum's group UK', which is a network of doctor mums providing peer-to-peer support, advice, and guidance on a whole breadth of work and life related issues. Those in training can also seek support and guidance from their deanery's professional support unit.

Thirdly, you should take the initiative to build networks that can drive change. Through collaboration, you can create supportive spaces to enable and facilitate each other to thrive. If you see a gap in your work environment for something that may help you or your peers, create a society, or initiative that aims to address it. This not only allows you to solve a problem but also creates a network with like-minded individuals, which in turn will create momentum and increase personal motivation. Inspired by the Women in Surgery Conference, Miss Sathanathan, one of the authors of this chapter, went on to create her own surgical society, Essex Surgical Girls, as a support system for herself and her peers who were applying to Core Surgical Training. Although it started small, today this has evolved into a much bigger organisation that supports a whole community of aspiring female core trainees. You will find that influencing others positively as you grow will not only compound your sense of confidence and success but also help boost your portfolio and professional growth.

In terms of addressing some of the stark inequalities we see between men and women within surgery, there is a dire need to include men in the conversation. In a study of over 300 surgeons across Europe, 72% of women report having suffered or witnessed gender abuse. However, worryingly, only 17% of male surgeons said they had witnessed gender discrimination at work (24). From these statistics, education about what is appropriate and inappropriate behaviour is necessary. There is potential to include this in our curriculums at both a university level and postgraduate level to effect the drastic change that is needed. Furthermore, we need to integrate these ideas into the mainstream conversations that are happening in surgical departments, such as in monthly audit meetings. It is paramount that sexual discrimination is recognised as an important ethical issue, which doctors have a moral obligation to recognise and object to (25). Male or female, it is important to engage, learn, and be a part of the conversation.

One of the biggest problems we face currently within the speciality is the need for safe, anonymous escalation pathways for surgeons who are experiencing bullying, undermining, and harassment within the workplace. If the goal is justice, the method must be a transparent, accountable, and working justice system to address the problems highlighted. There are organisations working on this, including the recently commissioned Working Party on Sexual Misconduct in Surgery and the initiative called Surviving in Scrubs, which aims to tackle misogyny within healthcare. We must continue to initiate, support, and promote this work and channel our own experiences to drive change.

If you have witnessed or been subject to something unacceptable that has made you uncomfortable in the workplace, it is important you process it. Seek counsel and advice from peers, seniors, mentors, and the groups and organisations mentioned in this chapter, firstly to gain a wider perspective on the situation and secondly to enlist support if you decide to take it further. Until our escalation pathways become more robust, it is worth doing a little bit of research into the most strategic and appropriate escalation pathway in your situation, and you should try to divulge the information to somebody that is trustworthy or has the power to effect change. Escalation options include your educational supervisor, college tutor, guardian for safe working, departmental lead, and educational deanery (directly or via the GMC survey).

SUMMARY OF HELPFUL STRATEGIES
- Seek counsel from seniors.
- Find at least one mentor and stay in regular communication with this individual.
- Take leadership and networking opportunities, especially those that will enable you to drive change.
- Understand and become familiar with escalation pathways in your department and institution.
- Be aware of the organisations that you can reach out to for support
- Aim to collaborate rather than compete with peers.
- When dealing with a difficult situation, take some time to think and process and liaise with those you trust before acting.

Conclusion

It is important that as a community of surgeons and aspiring surgeons, we seek to understand the multitude of challenges faced by women in surgery and continue to ameliorate our workplace environment in a way that facilitates women to thrive, flourish, and put forth their best work.

The motivation to endure, advocate, and drive change does not always reach us when we are vehemently occupied with our own career progression, but we must remember that surgery is no ordinary career. It is an extraordinary career for extraordinary individuals and the rewarding nature of the work we do knows no bounds.

We must choose to be brave, stay within this speciality, fight to navigate healthy career paths for ourselves with our personal goals, and continue striving to create a better work environment for those that come after us.

References

1. Royal College of Surgeons. Women in Surgery. www.rcseng.ac.uk/careers-in-surgery/women-in-surgery/statistics/.
2. Trinh LN, O'Rorke E, Mulcahey MK. Factors Influencing Female Medical Students' Decision to Pursue Surgical Specialties: A Systematic Review. J Surg Educ. 2021 May;78(3):836–49.
3. Park J, et al. Why Are Women Deterred from General Surgery Training? Am J Surg. 2005;(190):141–6.
4. Barnes KL, McGuire L, Dunivan G, Sussman AL, McKee R. Gender Bias Experiences of Female Surgical Trainees. J Surg Educ. 2019 Nov;76(6):e1–14.
5. Anderson M, Goldman RH. Occupational Reproductive Hazards for Female Surgeons in the Operating Room: A Review. JAMA Surg. 2020;155(3):243–9.
6. Lim WH, Wong C, Jain SR, Ng CH, Tai CH, Kamala Devi M, et al. The Unspoken Reality of Gender Bias in Surgery: A Qualitative Systematic Review. PLoS One. 2021;16(2 February).
7. Wallis CJ, Ravi B, Coburn N, Nam RK, Detsky AS, Satkunasivam R. Comparison of Postoperative Outcomes Among Patients Treated by Male and Female Surgeons: A Population Based Matched Cohort Study. BMJ (Online). 2017;359.
8. Giantini Larsen AM, Pories S, Parangi S, Robertson FC. Barriers to Pursuing a Career in Surgery: An Institutional Survey of Harvard Medical School Students. Ann Surg. 2021;273(6).
9. Sarsons H. Interpreting Signals in the Labor Market: Evidence from Medical Referrals. Mimeo. 2019.
10. Whitaker M. The Surgical Personality: Does It Exist? Ann R Coll Surg Engl. 2018;100(1).
11. Ali A, et al. Factors Influencing Career Choice Among Medical Students Interested in Surgery. Curr Surg. 2003;210–3.
12. Saalwachter AR, Freischlag JA, Sawyer RG, Sanfey HA. Part-Time Training in General Surgery: Results of a Web-Based Survey. Arch Surg. 2006 Oct;141(10):977–82.
13. Royal College of Surgeons England. Less Than Full Time Training. www.rcsed.ac.uk/professional-support-development-resources/career-support/return-to-work/less-than-full-time-training.
14. Möller MG, Elseth A, Sumra H, Riner AN. Time Out! We Must Address Fertility Preservation for Surgical Trainees. Am J Surg. 2022 Mar;223(3):594–5.
15. Stack SW, Jagsi R, Biermann JS, Lundberg GP, Law KL, Milne CK, et al. Childbearing Decisions in Residency: A Multicenter Survey of Female Residents. Acad Med. 2020 Oct 16;95(10):1550–7.

16. Phillips EA, Nimeh T, Braga J, Lerner LB. Does a Surgical Career Affect a Woman's Childbearing and Fertility? A Report on Pregnancy and Fertility Trends Among Female Surgeons. J Am Coll Surg. 2014 Nov;219(5):944–50.

17. Rangel EL, Castillo-Angeles M, Easter SR, Atkinson RB, Gosain A, Hu YY, et al. Incidence of Infertility and Pregnancy Complications in US Female Surgeons. JAMA Surg. 2021;156(10):905–15.

18. Phillips EA, Nimeh T, Braga J, Lerner LB. Does a Surgical Career Affect a Woman's Childbearing and Fertility? A Report on Pregnancy and Fertility Trends Among Female Surgeons. J Am Coll Surg. 2014 Nov;219(5):944–50.

19. The Royal College of Surgeons of England. An Independent Review on Diversity and Inclusion for the Royal College of Surgeons of England an Exciting Call for Radical Change. 2021 Mar.

20. Jadi J, Shaughnessy E, Barry L, Reyna C, Tsai S, Downs-Canner SM, & Myers, S (2023). Outcomes of a Pilot Virtual Mentorship Program for Medical Students Interested in Surgery. Am J Surg. 2022 Jul;225(2):229–33. https://doi:10.1016/j.amjsurg.2022.07.004.

21. ASiT. The ASiT Mentoring Scheme. www.asit.org/resources/asit-mentoring-scheme/the-asit-mentoring-scheme/res1131.

22. Gargiulo DA, Hyman NH, Hebert JC, Kirton O, Gawande A, Tseng J, et al. Women in Surgery: Do We Really Understand the Deterrents? Arch Surg. 2006;141.

23. Fleming S, Fisher R. Sexual Assault in Surgery: A Painful Truth. Bull R Coll Surg Engl. 2021;103(6).

24. New Survey Shines Light on Prejudice and Inequality in Colorectal Surgery | European Society of Coloproctology [Internet]. [cited 2022 Dec 30]. Available from: www.escp.eu.com/news/2398-new-survey-shines-light-on-prejudice-and-inequality-in-colorectal-surgery.

25. Mello MM, Jagsi R. Standing Up Against Gender Bias and Harassment – A Matter of Professional Ethics. N Engl J Med. 2020;382(15).

chapter seventeen

International Medical Graduates – Planning to a Move to the UK

Muhammad Talha, Muhammad Salik,
and Anokha Oomman Joseph

British surgical training is world-renowned and produces world-class surgeons. Pursuing a career in surgery in the United Kingdom (UK) as an international medical graduate (IMG) is a challenge. In this chapter, we aim to guide you on how to overcome these challenges and give you the best chance to get into training.

The first step is committing to the process of moving to the UK to pursue training. This will take deep reflection and consideration of all your available options. In general, training in the UK is considered to be rigorous and meritocratic. However, it is also one of the longest training programmes in the world for surgery. You may have other considerations, such as language, family ties, or finances.

Once you have decided, the next step is to get registration with the General Medical Council (GMC), the regulator for doctors in the UK. GMC registration is a mandatory requirement to be able to work as a doctor and the route you choose depends on your circumstances and your level of training. There are four routes for you to pursue if you want to practice medicine in the UK.

- Professional and Linguistic Assessments Board (PLAB)
- Applying for registration using sponsorship
- Acceptable postgraduate qualifications
- Relevant European qualification

Route 1: PLAB

The Professional and Linguistic Assessments Board (PLAB) exam is the licensing exam to get GMC registration (1). Prior to sitting the PLAB, you will need to demonstrate your competency in the English language by sitting the International English Language Testing System (IELTS) or the Occupational

DOI: 10.1201/9781003350422-18

English Test (OET), both of which are accepted by the GMC (2). These exams are valid for two years, and you will need to pass your PLAB exams in this period. IELTS tests your overall ability to communicate in the English language, whereas OET tests your ability to communicate in English in a healthcare setting (2).

The PLAB comprises two parts: Part 1 is an MCQ-based theory exam with 180 single-best-answer questions. Part 2 is a role-playing-based clinical competency exam. You will need to pass both these exams to be granted GMC registration. As it is an entry-level exam, it covers the whole of medicine at the level of completion of your medical degree.

Preparation for Part 1 of the PLAB can take an average of three months depending on your circumstance. We recommend subscribing to a question bank and practising as many questions as possible.

PLAB 2 is an objective, structured clinical examination (OSCE). It is conducted only in the UK at present. PLAB 2 is an OSCE-based exam which is conducted only in the UK at present. It has a heavy focus on ethics, communication skills, and professionalism. Dr Aman Arora's PLAB 2 communications skills resources (including online course, audiobook, and live course) are a great resource to improve your interpersonal and consultation skills. The OSCE has 16 stations, which last eight minutes each, where you will be asked to do a mock consultation.

This exam requires a lot of practice, and we highly recommend that you attend a PLAB 2 preparation course run (e.g. Swammy, Samson, Common Stations, or Aspire). It does not matter which provider you choose as the content of these courses is similar. The key here is to get a feel for the nature of the examination and the British way of answering questions. Doing mock exams with the PLAB 2 exam format is important for time management. You should do these once you feel adequately prepared.

United Kingdom Medical Licensing Assessment

The United Kingdom Medical Licensing Assessment (UKMLA) is the proposed exam to replace PLAB exams in 2024–2025.

This exam will consist of two parts: the Applied Knowledge Test (AKT), which will comprise 150 to 200 single-best-answer questions, and the Clinical and Professional Skills Assessment (CPSA), which will be a practical OSCE-based exam (3).

Anyone who wishes to practise in the UK will have to take this exam. Both UK graduates, as well as IMGs, will have to sit the same standardised exam and pass it to be considered fit to practise medicine in the UK and get GMC registration. The purpose of the UKMLA will be to ensure that both patients and employers have confidence in doctors working in the UK regardless of where they were trained and educated (3).

Route 2: Applying for Registration Using Sponsorship

In order to apply through the sponsorship route, you will need to demonstrate that you possess the experience, knowledge, and skills needed to work as a fully registered medical doctor in the UK.

There is a list of sponsors that have been pre-approved by the GMC. If you can satisfy the requirements for the sponsored post and can secure a job after successfully interviewing, you can apply for a certificate of sponsorship, which you will need for the GMC registration.

If your sponsor is not on the GMC pre-approved list, then you cannot apply using sponsorship and will need to consider one of the other routes (4).

Route 3: Acceptable Postgraduate Qualifications

It is possible to apply for GMC registration using acceptable postgraduate qualifications such as membership in the Royal College of Surgeons (MRCS) (5). MRCS is a two-part intercollegiate exam. It is organised by the Royal College of Surgeons of England, Royal College of Surgeons of Edinburgh, Royal College of Physicians and Surgeons of Glasgow, and Royal College of Surgeons in Ireland. You will need to provide a letter from the college where you passed the exam confirming your membership.

Part A of the MRCS is an MCQ-based theoretical exam, and Part B is a clinical OSCE-based surgical skills exam. You need to allocate around six months to prepare for this. The exam can be taken internationally in a few different countries listed on the Royal College of Surgeons website.

MRCS is a requirement to complete Core Surgical Training. You cannot progress to higher surgical training without passing the MRCS exams. Coming via this route has the added benefit of meeting that requirement while at the same time getting GMC registration. Once you have the GMC registration, you will be eligible to apply for and work in the UK in middle-grade surgical roles as a surgical registrar.

If you are currently in or have finished surgical training in your home country, then applying for GMC registration with the acceptable postgraduate qualification route might make more sense. Once you are in the UK, you can apply for higher surgical training and skip Core Surgical Training.

The other acceptable postgraduate exam is the Joint Surgical Colleges' Fellowship Examination (JSCFE) (6). This is a much harder exam compared to the MRCS and one that is similar to the exam normally given at the end of higher surgical training in the UK. The JSCFE is aimed at international surgeons and is held by all four royal surgical colleges (England, Edinburgh, Glasgow, and Ireland).

Success in both JSCFE Section 1 and Section 2 will allow affiliation to one of the four surgical royal colleges of Great Britain and Ireland and, from January 2023, introduce the use of the post-nominal IntFRCS (College). This post-nominal has been revised as it differentiates the qualification from the Intercollegiate Speciality Examination (6).

At present, you can apply for GMC registration once you have passed the JSCFE as it is listed as an acceptable post-graduate qualification.

Route 4: Relevant European Qualification

The GMC accepts relevant European qualifications from countries with both the primary degree and some approved specialist qualifications listed on the GMC website (7). If you have this, you can apply for GMC registration.

Special Considerations for IMGs

Applying for Jobs

Jobs are advertised online and can be accessed via websites such as NHS Jobs and Trac Jobs. Applications are submitted through the same websites. You do not need to make separate applications for all jobs, as you can import your data from your previous applications to your next application and just make suitable changes as you go along. Jobs in Scotland can be accessed via a separate website, NHS Scotland Jobs (8). Do not miss out on these jobs as Scotland is a whole another country, and they have the same shortage of highly skilled professionals as the rest of England, Wales, and Northern Ireland.

It is very difficult to start with a training post as your first job because often the requirements needed for these are difficult to get if you are not already working in the NHS. It is advisable to start with a non-training job and get to know the system. During this time, you can prepare your portfolio and get ready for the next round of national interviews. There is a shortage of highly skilled professionals like doctors. The NHS is always recruiting.

Jobs are advertised all year long. However, there is a significant increase in vacancies around August, as a lot of speciality training jobs start at that time creating a workforce vacuum. This pattern is also repeated around February for a similar reason.

As you are an IMG, it takes time to understand the application process and what it is asking from you. It is important to be truthful in the application. Lying on your application is a probity issue and may create problems for future job applications. Make sure you have read the specifications of the job and ensure your application contains the relevant information. You need to keep working towards improving your CV. It can take several months and hundreds of applications until you finally get an interview. You will notice with time your understanding of the application process improves, and your CV becomes polished. For one of the authors of this chapter, the first interview invite came after six months and 300+ applications. The second one came two to three weeks after the first, and the author secured the job offer after his second interview.

Preparing for Job Interviews

Treat your interview like an exam. Preparation is key. There is a fantastic interview book titled *Medical Interviews*, written by Olivier Picard, which deals with medical interview questions in a very comprehensive way. Blogs on the internet and IMG groups on social networking sites are very helpful. We have listed some useful resources at the end of this chapter. Finally, mock interview practice with someone who is working in the NHS or who has recently been successful in an NHS interview is a great way to prepare.

Accepting the Job Offer

Once you have been offered a job, it is important to make sure you clarify a few things. You have to ask them if they certify maintenance for you and your dependent (dependents are your family; i.e. partner and kids). If they do, you do not need to show personal funds in your visa application. However, if they do not then you need to show sufficient funds to support yourself and your family for one month in the UK until you start getting paid. In this scenario, it is better suited that you come to the UK before your family. You can then apply for your family's visa after two to three months, once you have saved some money in your bank to show that you can support your family.

Visa

Short-Term – Visiting Visa

You must have sufficient funds to support yourself during your stay. If you are coming to the UK, the anecdotal advice is to have at least two to three times the savings compared to your expected expenses in the UK. For example, if you are applying for a ten-day visa, and you expect your expense to be £1,000, then your savings should be £2,000–3,000.

It is wise to plan early and start saving up accordingly for the journey. You can also choose to have someone sponsor your visit instead. The sponsor has to be a close family member, like one of your parents. They have to give you a signed letter of support mentioning how much funds they will be giving you for your trip and you have to attach their bank statement as evidence of those funds.

You can find the official visa guidance on the UK Visa and Immigration (UK VI) website. It is important you check this, as the requirements are updated regularly (9). Typically, the documents that are required for a visit visa for an exam include your passport, an employment letter and a no objection certificate (NOC) from your current employer, a police character certificate, your exam booking confirmation email, a bank statement or sponsorship letter as evidence of funds available to you for your visit, and your return ticket with accommodation booking in the UK for the duration of your stay.

Whilst in the UK for the PLAB 2, you should make the most of your time and try to get a clinical attachment or courses, such as ALS, under your belt.

Long-Term – Health and Care Worker Visa

Once you have a job and GMC registration, you will need to apply for health and care worker visa (previously known as Tier 2 visa) (10).

This visa is aimed at medical professionals, who can come to or stay in the UK to fill an eligible post in the NHS.

You must have a job offer from an approved UK employer, such as the NHS, before you apply for a health and care worker visa. Approved employers are also known as sponsors, they will be sponsoring your stay in the UK. Your employer will check that you meet the eligibility requirements and provide you with a certificate of sponsorship. This is an electronic record and not a physical document. It will have a reference number, which you will need for your visa application. You must apply for your visa within three months of getting your certificate of sponsorship.

Indefinite Leave to Remain

You will need to stay in the UK for five years to qualify for indefinite leave to remain (ILR). Once you have ILR you will become a permanent resident in the UK and do not need to apply or renew your visa every few years. You can apply for a British passport one year after getting ILR (11).

Useful Resources

There are many online blogs and Facebook pages that have useful resources for IMGs to help plan your move to the UK. We have listed a few of these here:

1. Salik Surgery Series   https://saliksurgeryseries.com
2. Naseer's Journey   https://naseersjourney.com/
3. Omar Guidelines   http://omarsguidelines.blogspot.com/
4. Road to UK   https://roadtouk.com/
5. The Savvy IMG   https://thesavvyimg.co.uk/
6. International Medical Graduates (IMGs) in the UK – Facebook page

Active pages have the most members and should be the most helpful. These pages are free to join and contain useful help and information.

One of the authors of this chapter, Muhammad Salik, maintains a website called Salik Surgery Series (12), which focuses on applying for jobs in the UK, interview preparation, surgical portfolio building, and other aspects of life as an IMG and a surgical trainee.

References

1. GMCRegistrationandLicensing.www.gmc-uk.org/registration-and-licensing/join-the-register/plab.
2. GMC Registration and IELTS. www.gmc-uk.org/registration-and-licensing/join-the-register/before-you-apply/evidence-of-your-knowledge-of-english/using-your-ielts-certificate.
3. GMC. GMC Medical Licensing Assessment. www.gmc-uk.org/education/medical-licensing-assessment.
4. GMC Registration Using Sponsorship. www.gmc-uk.org/registration-and-licensing/join-the-register/before-you-apply/list-of-approved-sponsoring-bodies.
5. GMC.AcceptablePostGraduateQualification.www.gmc-uk.org/registration-and-licensing/join-the-register/before-you-apply/acceptable-postgraduate-qualifications.
6. Joint Surgical Colleges Fellowship Examination. www.jscfe.co.uk/Content/content.aspx.
7. GMC Relevant European Qualifications. www.gmc-uk.org/-/media/documents/factsheet–international-apps–relevant-european-qualifications-list –dc11865_pdf-78131156.pdf.
8. NHS Scotland Jobs. https://jobs.scot.nhs.uk.
9. GMC. UK Visa and Immigration.
10. Gov.UK. Skilled Worker Visa. www.gov.uk/skilled-worker-visa.
11. British Citizenship. www.gov.uk/british-citizenship.
12. Muhammad Salik. Salik Surgical Series. https://saliksurgeryseries.com.

chapter eighteen

International Medical Graduates – Planning a Career in Surgery

Muhammad Salik, Muhammad Talha,
and Anokha Oomman Joseph

A career in surgery requires a lot of hard work. You will have to make personal sacrifices and work on your own time to improve your CV and build a good portfolio. It takes time to get used to the NHS system, living in a new country. As an IMG, there are extra layers of challenges to becoming a surgeon in the UK. Take one step at a time to avoid feeling overwhelmed by this journey. In this chapter, we will outline ways you can enter training and navigate a career in surgery as an IMG in the UK.

Making Opportunities

Once you have decided to become a surgeon, make yourself visible and available. Speak to seniors you are on shift with. Tell them your requirements – is it an audit or a publication you want? Do you need procedures for your logbook? Are you interested in going to theatre? Once everyone knows you are interested, they will make opportunities for you. It is then up to you to work hard and avail of every opportunity you can get.

One thing to keep in mind here is that it is very important to choose your projects wisely. Do not get involved in a big project which cannot finish in a defined period. You need to be mindful of time and get involved in projects that are likely to finish and get you the most marks in your portfolio.

Foundation Competencies and CREST Form

If you are not in a foundation programme, you will need a Certificate of Readiness to Enter Speciality Training (CREST) form to be signed in order to be eligible to apply for a training post (1). You can get it signed by any consultant you have worked with for three months or more. These are competencies equivalent to completion of foundation training in the UK.

DOI: 10.1201/9781003350422-19

Some consultants are happy to observe you on the job and sign you off if they find your performance satisfactory, whereas others will want you to collect formal evidence before they sign you off.

You should use the Horus e-portfolio program to collect evidence. Horus is the platform used by the foundation doctors in England to collect evidence for their foundation competencies, and therefore, it has all the sections needed for the CREST form. If your hospital does not provide this for free, you will need to get a subscription yourself. We recommend that you speak to the postgraduate office of the hospital in which you work and familiarise yourself with the foundation curriculum so that you can match your e-portfolio with those of foundation trainees.

Route to Surgical Training in the UK

Core Surgical Training (CST)

Following GMC registration, you can get a standalone foundation year 2 post (FY2), non-training jobs, or clinical development fellow posts in NHS preferably in surgery (2).

Many IMGs have already completed one to two years of postgraduate experience (including a house job) before coming to the UK, but this international experience is not officially recognised. In order to get onto the training pathway, you need to get your foundation competencies signed off first. Once you have your foundation competencies signed off, you can apply for Core Surgical Training.

There is an 18-month surgical experience limit for getting into Core Surgical Training. You will be classed as overqualified and will not be allowed to apply at CT1/ST1 level if you do a surgical job for more than 18 months post-graduation (not including your foundation training, internship, or house job). Opportunities to build a surgical portfolio are better in a surgical job; however, if you already have significant surgical experience, then it is important to avoid a surgical job so as to stay within the 18-month mark.

After completing Core Surgical Training and passing the MRCS exams you can apply for ST3 (3).

Skipping CST and Applying to Higher Surgical Training (HST)

Alternatively, you can skip CST in case you have exceeded the 18-month surgical experience limit, or you choose to go for speciality training directly. This pathway can be shorter or longer than the conventional CST pathway, depending on each individual. Some people get their

CST competencies with the Certificate of Readiness to Enter Higher Surgical Training (CREHST) form signed off in six months, and for some, it may take two to three years. This form can be downloaded from the Royal College of Surgeons (RCS) website, and it is a recognised alternative to confirm the competencies of CST. Furthermore, you will also need to complete your MRCS Part A and Part B exams before applying for HST.

Remember, it is not a race. Everyone has their own timeline. Work at your own pace, but remember that determination, perseverance, and hard work are key. All candidates taking the CREHST pathway previously would have gotten the Certificate of Eligibility of Specialist Registration – Combined Programme (CESR-CP). But since 2020, the GMC has confirmed that eligible doctors on the CESR-CP pathway will be awarded Certificate of Completion of Training (CCT) upon completion of training (4). Therefore, everyone completing HST in the UK will graduate with the same certificate, regardless of where they received their CST competencies from.

Certificate of Eligibility for Specialist Registration (CESR)

CESR allows doctors who have not completed a UK specialist training programme but have a combination of qualifications, training, and experience gained anywhere in the world, to be evaluated as part of an application for entry to the GMC Specialist Register. This pathway takes a long time (5). It is suitable for surgeons who have completed surgical training in their home country, passed the MRCS, and joined the NHS as a non-training middle grade after GMC registration. The experience they gained from their training abroad and non-training posts done in the UK will need to be demonstrated equivalence to surgeons who have achieved their competencies with a CCT. Equivalence demonstrated has to be to the current curriculum current at the time of application; following this, you will be awarded the CESR (5).

Conclusion

Give yourself time to adjust to a new way of life. You will need to adjust to your new role and responsibilities, a new country, and a new culture. Everyone is different and requires a different amount of time until they become comfortable in their new environment.

Take it easy, take it slow, progress in small steps, and when you feel ready, pick up the latest CST self-assessment document and start planning your portfolio development. Set clear goals and focus on achieving them.

Be mindful of the projects you take on and pick them wisely. Do not waste time on anything that will not help you in building the perfect portfolio. Speak to your seniors and other IMGs who have been successful in this journey for advice.

There are many ways in which you can pursue a career in surgery. Where you want to start will depend on your own individual experience.

References

1. Speciality Training Health Education England. Certificate of Readiness to Enter Speciality Training. https://specialtytraining.hee.nhs.uk/portals/1/Content/Resource%20Bank/Recruitment%20Documents/CREST%202021%20Reference%20Version.pdf.
2. Royal College of Surgeons of England. Surgery Entry Requirements. www.rcseng.ac.uk/careers-in-surgery/careers-support/what-is-surgery-like-as-a-career/entry-requirements-and-training/.
3. Royal College of Surgeons England. Career Paths in Surgery. www.rcseng.ac.uk/careers-in-surgery/trainees/foundation-and-core-trainees/surgery-career-paths/.
4. Tim Tonkin B. GMC Simplifies Access to CCT. www.bma.org.uk/news-and-opinion/gmc-simplifies-access-to-cct. 2020.
5. GMC. CESR Application. www.gmc-uk.org/registration-and-licensing/join-the-register/registration-applications/specialty-specific-guidance-for-cesr-and-cegpr/specialty-specific-guidance-for-cesr-in-general-surgery.

chapter nineteen

Dyslexia and Neurodiversity

Carol Leather

The aim of this chapter is to increase the understanding of dyslexia, discuss its impact on doctors in training, and suggest strategies for success. You may already have a diagnosis of dyslexia. Alternatively, you may be struggling with an aspect of work or with repeated failures in examinations, but be unaware of an underlying diagnosis of dyslexia. In either case, this chapter is for you. While the focus is on dyslexia, there are commonalities with other syndromes, such as dyspraxia and attention deficit disorder (ADD).

The chapter is split into three sections:

- Understanding Adult Dyslexia – a Brief Theoretical Outline
- The Assessment Process – What, When, Why, and How to Tell People
- Support for Examinations and the Workplace – Tips and Strategies

Understanding Adult Dyslexia – a Brief Theoretical Outline

Despite the recognition of dyslexia over 100 years ago, it is still an area of some controversy, particularly in adulthood. It is often misunderstood. This is not surprising and partially stems from the lack of consensus regarding the definition. Dyslexia is something of a conundrum because it is widely recognised as a reading and spelling difficulty. However, many dyslexic adults – in particular, professionals like doctors – may have developed their literacy skills to a competent level. Furthermore, the characteristics of dyslexic individuals vary. Some are articulate, and others struggle to find words. Some people are visual, and others are not. Some dyslexic people are successful, and others less so. It is these disparities that lead to confusion for both dyslexic individuals themselves and those around them. The heterogeneity of dyslexia in adulthood is predictable as dyslexia is developmental. We are all products of our environments, cultures, family life, educational opportunities, experiences, and personalities (1). The individuality and the complexity of dyslexia mean that understanding it and how it affects you as an individual is paramount.

DOI: 10.1201/9781003350422-20

Another reason for the misunderstanding of dyslexia is the dearth of research in adults. Most research has been limited to children or student populations and so is not relatable to the workplace. Further, the child focus in research has influenced definitions, limited the understanding of the impact in adulthood, and led to some interventions being inappropriate. The literacy skills of many dyslexic adults are competent, especially when aided by technology. Hence, in some workplace contexts, problems faced by dyslexic people are broader and include time management and memory recall (2, 3).

The Positive Impact of Dyslexia

Interestingly much of the research conducted on dyslexic adults in employment has focused on success attributes (4–6). Successful dyslexic adults are good problem-solvers. They have good reasoning skills and are often creative thinkers. The positive impact of being dyslexic is increased determination, perseverance, and high motivation. Furthermore, some experts argue that self-awareness and high job self-efficacy are other factors related to their success (7). Does this sound like you?

What Is Adult Dyslexia?

There are many definitions of dyslexia. Some are narrow in their scope, referring to difficulty acquiring literacy skills and difficulty with phonological processing (the ability to use the sounds in language to process the spoken and written words). This has led to the possibility of misdiagnosis and misunderstanding, particularly of those adults who have been described as 'literate' dyslexics (8). Medical students and doctors are usually in this category. They have developed their reading and spelling skills to a competent level but experience broader difficulties in domains, such as reading speed and comprehension, written expression, note-taking, clarity of communication, time management, memory, and organisation (2).

Researchers and practitioners are now adopting broader definitions such as that proposed by the British Dyslexia Association.

> Dyslexia is a specific learning difficulty that mainly affects the development of literacy and language-related skills. It is likely to be present at birth and to be lifelong in its effects. It is characterised by difficulties with phonological processing, rapid naming, working memory, processing speed and the automatic development of skills that may not match up to an individual's other cognitive abilities (9).

This definition includes cognitive processes, such as working memory and speed of processing; the measurement of both is generally required for a diagnosis. These account for the residual difficulties with reading speed and comprehension and memory recall.

Neurodiversity

The need for a clearer definition is also important because of the issue of comorbidity with other specific learning disabilities that come under the umbrella of neuro-developmental disabilities.

These include the following:

- Dyspraxia: problems with motor coordination, sequencing, planning difficulties
- Attention deficit/hyperactivity disorder (ADD and ADHD): difficulties with concentration
- Autistic spectrum disorder: social communication problems
- Dyscalculia: a problem with mathematical conceptualisation and calculation

While there is some similarity in the characteristics of these syndromes, the causes of each specific disability are different and have different neurological correlates. Rates of comorbidity between dyslexia and other disorders vary but it has been suggested that it is the rule rather than the exception.

To frame all these overlapping syndromes more positively, the umbrella term 'neurodiversity' has been adopted. This concept is seen as having more positive connotations. It includes a wide range of syndromes, and so there is a larger single voice for advocacy purposes. It also possibly allows for a more comfortable way to discuss what an individual might need to work well. It can, however, create even more confusion as there are no specific criteria for the diagnosis of neurodiversity, but there are distinguishing profiles for syndromes, such as dyslexia. Some people argue that each syndrome loses its distinct identity under the umbrella term, and even dilutes the support and increases misunderstanding. They prefer to be just dyslexic. In any event, the need for self-understanding and self-advocacy is important.

The Evidence for Dyslexia

As far back as 1999, Frith developed a framework to gain a better understanding of dyslexia across the lifespan, at biological, cognitive, and behavioural levels; this framework could be adopted across to cover various syndromes referred to here.

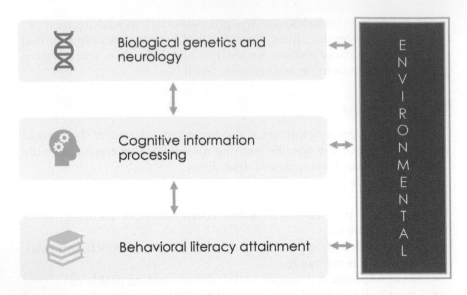

Figure 19.1 Frith's model of dyslexia.

Frith wrote,

> Defining dyslexia at a single level of explanation –
> biological, cognitive, or behavioural – will always lead
> to paradoxes. For a full understanding of dyslexia, we
> need to link together the three levels and consider
> the impact of cultural factors which can aggravate
> or ameliorate the condition. Consensus is emerging
> that dyslexia is a neurodevelopmental disorder with
> a biological origin, which impacts on speech process-
> ing with a wide range of clinical manifestations (10).

Frith also suggested that each of these levels interacts within the
individual and their environment, which accounts for the heterogeneity
amongst the population of dyslexic adults.

The *biological level* includes genetics and neurology. Genetics are evi-
denced in the plethora of family and twin studies. The development of
fMRI scans has meant that neurological differences between dyslexic and
non-dyslexic readers can be identified both at the structural and functional levels (11).

The *cognitive level* involves the processes that are associated with
acquiring information, including learning and reading and also with the

Dyslexia – Why Is It Presenting Itself Now?

Dyslexia can present itself at any time across the lifespan, but it is usually at times of transition or overload. The transition from GCSE to A-level where the teaching method changes can lead to unexpectedly poor results. Likewise, the move to university when independent self-directed learning makes demands on organisational skills can result in students feeling overloaded and result in poor performance at medical school. University to work is another transition into a new learning environment. People are diagnosed at any one of these times. Nevertheless, being able to put in more time, perhaps working through the night to get all the assignments in, means people continue to achieve their goals. However, when in the workplace, trying to revise for professional examinations is a very challenging task. There are not enough hours in the day or enough energy to revise and learn effectively. This is particularly true when there are increased family demands, young children, or older parents or even after a difficult day in the clinical setting. The result can be poor performance in an examination and/or burnout, as well as a huge loss of confidence. The time to find out a reason you have to work longer and harder than others should be before this happens. It may be time to seek advice.

The Assessment Process – What, When, Why, and How to Tell People

There are many reasons for seeking an assessment. Sometimes it is driven by the individual. They have often wondered why they are different. Sometimes it is prompted by a family member, a friend, or a colleague being diagnosed. More frequently now in the medical profession, it is suggested by educational supervisors or more senior doctors trying to be supportive when there has been unexpected poor performance in examinations.

An assessment should be an informative, positive experience. If it is recommended by others, it is important that you are comfortable with the idea. There is often some pressure to have an assessment. However, if you have never thought about it, and especially if there are cultural implications, a positive diagnosis can be a shock and take a while to come to terms with. It can then be counterproductive. Being well prepared for an assessment, such as knowing something about dyslexia and the process, can help. However, going online to seek information is not always the best way, as there are a great many negative texts – long lists of all the difficulties people might experience – and it can be overwhelming. Ideally, it is best to talk to someone who can explain what it all entails. The professional support unit or the individual support team at your deanery or occupational health should be able to help. You should be able to seek advice and maintain confidentiality if you wish.

Steps to Assessment

Checklists

Completing a checklist can be helpful as the starting point for consideration for further investigation. One of the most reliable is the adult checklist (12). However, while it is based on thorough research, it is a subjective tool. It is a guide rather than a definitive assessment tool. There is the possibility of both false positives and false negatives. Individuals can respond to the questions in a way that they think they should answer rather than an accurate reflection of what they do. Nevertheless, checklists are a good indicator, and they do help in the preparation process. There are also some computer-based screening tests available online, but like the checklists, they can produce false negatives.

It might be that a checklist or screening result may provide enough of an explanation for an individual, and they do not need to seek further assessment. There is little doubt, however, that the formal diagnosis provides much more information, particularly about where strengths lie. A formal diagnosis is required if any adjustments are to be made in the workplace or in examinations.

There are two routes to formal diagnosis: either through referral from occupational health (OH), human resources (HR), or a professional service unit (PSU) or by seeking a private assessment. Assessments for dyslexia should be conducted by trained educational and occupational psychologists or teachers who have specialist training. A private assessment means there is total confidentiality. You do not have to mention anything to anyone until you feel like they need to know. However, a private assessment can be expensive, and it is important that you do some research into finding an appropriately experienced person who offers the service at a reasonable cost. Being referred through OH, HR, or the PSU means that more people are involved, but confidentiality should remain within your control. You are likely to be referred to a recommended assessor. It also means that there is a support system post-diagnosis.

The Diagnostic Assessment

Any diagnosis, be it medical, psychological, or educational, should inform, explain, and effect a change. It should not just be a labelling process (11). The aim of an assessment is to gather information regarding people's abilities, both strengths and weaknesses. It should outline their educational achievements and literacy skill attainment, determine any inconsistencies, and provide an explanation for these. The diagnosis, be it dyslexia or another specific learning difficulty, is the result of a process of differential evaluation and clinical judgement.

Historically, diagnostic assessments have been conducted in person, where the assessor can more readily observe both verbal and non-verbal behaviour. However there has been a move towards online assessment. Some of the measures of assessment have been adapted to deal with this different administration and are seen as reliable; however, some psychologists would argue that in a face-to-face interaction, the building of rapport is easier and the observation of the person's behaviour when completing the tests is very important.

The Assessment Process

A diagnostic assessment includes the administration of measures of intellectual ability, cognitive processing, and literacy attainment. If other areas of difficulty arise or are mentioned by the person, additional testing, such as for numeracy, or checklists for other specific learning difficulties may be administered.

The measures of intellectual ability are important in predicting what people can achieve. Good intellectual abilities are likely to be part of the explanation for dyslexia not having been noticed previously.

The measures of cognitive processing include tests of phonological processing, rapid naming, working memory, and symbolic processing speed. These underlie the development of literacy skills and therefore impact reading, writing, and spelling attainment. Rapid naming is associated with fluent comprehension and word finding. Weak verbal short-term memory is likely to affect remembering lists of instructions, telephone numbers, and PINs. These cognitive processing skills are related to both working memory and executive functioning processes and, therefore, can also affect time management and organisation skills. It is deficits in these processes that can explain any inconsistencies in performance and result in a diagnosis.

Measures of literacy attainment include tests of single-word reading, reading speed, reading comprehension, spelling, and writing speed. Many adults working at a high level, such as doctors, will have developed their literacy skills to a competent level. However, when measured, it is apparent that there are residual difficulties with reading fluency and comprehension, as well as with writing speed. While many people comment that they must re-read to understand or they read slowly, they are not aware of how effortful the reading process is for them. Unlike other people, they have not developed their literacy skills to an automatic level.

At the end of the assessment, whatever the outcome, the results should be explained, and ideally, a diagnosis should be provided. The diagnosis may be something of a surprise, and people need to be given the time to ask questions and hopefully feel that it was a positive experience on which they can build. They should leave feeling better informed and know what is available to enable them to move forward. An assessment report is provided and should include test details, results, and conclusions. It should also make recommendations for skill development, assistive technology, and adjustments to the workplace. Preferably the assessment report should come in two sections: The first part has all the personal information and test results for individual perusal. The second part is a summary of the assessment and focuses on the recommendations, which can be shared with supervisors, colleagues, and employers.

Coming to Terms with a Diagnosis

However prepared people are, the actual diagnosis can generate a range of emotions. Even for those that were diagnosed in childhood, it can be a surprise as they may have thought they had overcome their dyslexia because their reading and writing skills were passable, and they have not been sufficiently aware of the impact as an adult.

For many people knowing what is causing the problem is a huge relief as it shows they are not incompetent. They have a reason as to why things have been so hard. The results can give them more confidence in their abilities, which may have been subsumed in the effort of learning and working. It can increase their confidence and their motivation.

There are some people who take a pragmatic stance. The diagnosis provides them with some extra time during examinations, and that is all they need to pass. They then move on.

For other people, the diagnosis is not so welcome; it brings with it confusion, denial, and disbelief: *How can I be dyslexic when I can read and write? How can I have suddenly become dyslexic?* This disbelief is sometimes compounded by others too: *You can't be dyslexic if you have been to university.* People can be frustrated by the identification of problems that they have always just gotten on with. Likewise, there can be anger that it was not diagnosed at school. Sometimes there comes a sense of loss, of what might have been if they had known earlier. Some people feel ashamed and see it as a disability or are worried that others will see it as such. There can be fear for the future. They are concerned that it will affect their promotion or their career progression, and so there can be a loss of motivation.

There is no doubt that even those people who take it positively will consider some of the more negative responses. The diagnosis can change how you see yourself for a while. When you are diagnosed at this stage, you should be commended as you have been studying and working with an unacknowledged condition that has placed you at a disadvantage in a very literate world. Despite this, you have achieved a great deal and can now go even further. You are the same person as before the diagnosis, just better informed.

Disclosure

One of the big questions following the diagnosis is disclosure. Should you tell people you are dyslexic? Whom should you tell, and when should you say something? Historically, disclosure rates have been low for fear of being misunderstood or thought stupid or incompetent (13). Amongst doctors, fear of discrimination is another concern (14). However, failure to disclose is associated with a lack of success in both clinical and written examinations (15). Furthermore, as the recognition of dyslexia increases, more people are happier about telling people. The positives of disclosure are ideally greater understanding at work and the provision of reasonable adjustments at work. The most common adjustment and one that people often seek an assessment for, and indeed benefit from, is extra time in an examination. The negative aspect is that people may see you differently, and there is a fear of stigma. This can be counteracted by considering what to say and how to present yourself.

It is a very personal decision, and unsurprisingly, peoples' approaches are very different. Some people are very keen to tell everyone all about it. Others are reticent and only bring it up when things go wrong. Some people mention it when they have been complimented for doing a good job: *I am so glad I passed that exam because I am dyslexic and exams are not the way I demonstrate my knowledge.*

The best time to tell people is when you feel comfortable and as confident as you can about it. When going to a new rotation or placement, it may be best to leave it to a second meeting so that people see you as an individual first, not a dyslexic. It is important to know what to say, how dyslexia affects you, and what you do about it: *I am dyslexic, which for me means I might need a bit of extra time to settle in. Once I am familiar with everything, I do a good job;* or *I always make notes to ensure I get it right;* or *if I have the speech-to-text software, I will be able to do the admin more quickly.* In summary, try to keep it short, simple, positive, and solution-focused.

Another thing to consider is what to say if supervisors ask what they can do to support you. Asking for what you need to work well and why it helps you gives them more confidence in you. For example, you may say, *I need a bit of extra time to learn the new IT system or even clinical procedures, but once I have learned it, I never forget;* or *I need to take notes so that I don't miss anything;* or *I like to ask more questions to clarify something.*

Support for Examinations and the Workplace – Tips and Strategies

The diagnostic report should make evidence-based recommendations regarding the support you need. There are three strands that can be useful to explore both for exams and in the workplace. They are as follows:

- *Skill development:* Developing the skills you need will improve your performance; specialist coaching is usually recommended for this.
- *Technological and practical aids:* These can make life easier. Assistive technology – speech-to-text packages, such as Dragon Dictation, or text-to-speech packages, such as Claro or Texthelp Read&Write Gold – can help with literacy accuracy. However, increasingly, both Google and Microsoft 365 have voice recognition and text-to-speech functions on their platforms. Practical aids can be as simple as more filing space to be better organised or whiteboards to help plan and recall information.
- *Adjustments to the workplace or training:* This includes extra time in exams or extended training. Some usually admin-related tasks in the workplace may need to be adjusted.

Reasonable Adjustments

Dyslexia can be considered a disability for the purposes of the Equality Act 2010. This means that organisations are obliged to make reasonable adjustments. The response to this has often been a one-size-fits-all approach, but what is reasonable for one person is not necessarily true of another. Therefore, adjustments should be evidence-based and tailored to the individual. The evidence is often provided in the diagnostic report. Having said that, the most important and common adjustment for any dyslexic individual is time – extra time to learn and develop new skills and effective personalised strategies to address the different ways of processing; extra time in written examinations to mitigate reading fluency difficulties; extra time to formulate an answer either in a viva or at work due to the word-finding difficulties; extra time to produce written work for processing and to allow for planning and proofreading.

Adjustments in Examinations

Most examination boards will send a list of the adjustments available for the examination on the receipt of the diagnostic report.

Written examinations adjustments include the following:

- Twenty-five per cent extra time. More time can be granted based on the recommendations in the report.
- A paper-based examination rather than taking the exam online. This allows the individual to annotate and interpret the question more effectively.
- Sitting the examination in a separate room. This allows for reading the question aloud and avoiding being distracted or distracting others. This also benefits ADD candidates.

- Paper to jot down ideas. This is particularly useful if the exam is online.
- An appropriately sized font.
- Coloured paper or backgrounds if required.

Adjustments in Vivas, Clinical, or Practical Examinations

Extra time may be given if there is quite a large reading component in these exams, but there are fewer adjustments. However, the following is good practice:

- Having paper and pencil to hand
- Being given the time to jot down relevant information
- Allowing candidates to ask for repetition and clarification and giving them more time to respond
- Allowing time to formulate an answer

Some medical examination boards will also consider allowing candidates to re-sit an examination more often, discounting previous attempts when there has been a late diagnosis, acknowledging that they have been at a disadvantage.

Adjustments in the Workplace

Adjustments to the workplace are made on the recommendations in the diagnostic report and sometimes on work-based assessments which are conducted by Occupation Health or, in the UK, Access to Work. The latter is a government-funded scheme.

The adjustments include the following:

- Extra time to complete documentation – ring-fenced time for administrative work
- Extra time in training and on equipment and techniques
- Assistive technology – voice recognition, text-to-speech
- Use of two computer screens
- Flexibility around working hours

These adjustments are granted based on individual needs and the demands of the job. Some might only be needed temporarily while you settle into your job role and develop task-specific expertise. In these cases, some adjustments are made on an informal basis and are a result of good communication between supervisors and their dyslexic trainees.

Coaching

Specialist coaching is now widely recommended following a diagnostic assessment; increasingly, it is seen as an important intervention that improves performance and self-efficacy (16). As with psychologists, coaching should be provided by specialist dyslexia coaches who have experience working with doctors.

The aim of coaching is to increase your understanding of dyslexia, your abilities and how you learn and work most effectively, and how to self-advocate.

> When I am performing a complicated surgical procedure, I find it very hard to talk/to describe what I am doing at that point in time, I am almost in another zone. I know what I am doing is correct – I am often complimented on doing a good job but when my consultant asks me to describe what the procedure is as I do it, it starts to go wrong. I have asked if I can tell him after the operation is complete.
>
> **(MRCS trainee, personal communication)**

As suggested earlier, dyslexia can be simply defined as a language-processing difference. It can be hard to multitask with words, so there is cognitive overload. The working memory does not work so efficiently, then it might be best to do one thing at a time, as indicated in the previous quote. It is also important with experience and practice tasks become more automatic, multitasking can become possible (1). Furthermore, if you plan and prepare using your executive functioning processes, it mitigates the working memory inefficiency (2, 3).

The coaching should be led by you to address your challenges and to enable you to ask for what you need to work well. This is especially important in the workplace. It should also help to develop specific skills,

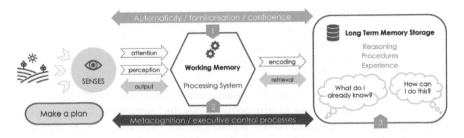

Figure 19.3 Information processing model.

such as planning and time management, efficient literacy skills if necessary, presenting to others, and of course, strategies for memory, revision, and examinations.

Strategies for Revision – The Four Ms

Make It Manageable

Plan and break the revision into chunks. Planning is an executive function process, and it is something we do both automatically and deliberately. It is one of the keys to success as it usually leads to a better outcome. For example, we tend to plan a party or a holiday. It also improves cognitive functioning and, therefore, performance by relieving cognitive overload. If we think about what we are doing in advance, we are more likely to complete the task more efficiently. For example, as a doctor, you may read patient notes in advance, so you know something about them and what needs to be done before seeing them.

However, planning can take time and does not always work; often, a day's to-do list is not completed and revision plans are not achieved. If this happens, then it is likely that the goals were unrealistic, and it is more positive to look at what you have achieved and how effective it was rather than overfocusing on what has not been done. Then just reset the plan. It was the plan that failed, not you. Furthermore, there is plenty of research demonstrating people achieve more with a plan than without one. It focuses attention especially if you work to short goals, working for 30 minutes and then taking a small break to reboot your concentration. It is good practice to keep a log of what you have covered over the day or week.

Tips for effective planning include making it realistic, fun, and flexible; having a variety of different activities, such as making brief notes, drawing and annotating diagrams, and doing questions; and having a variety of resources (e.g. books, webinars, YouTube, group study). It must also include ring-fenced time for rest and relaxation. A tired brain does not work well, and so the revision is less useful (17).

Make Revision Meaningful

Learning and revision are much more effective if you reprocess it into a format that you find more accessible and if you build on what you already know. Before looking at a topic, think about and try and recall as much as you can, then you can identify gaps and fill them. Also, look at the relevance of the topic – why are you required to learn it? Look at the high-yield topics – why are these so important? – and ensure you know these well.

Make It Multisensory

All learning is better if it is learned or revisited by utilising all your senses. See it, hear it, say it, do it. This is the reason that most doctors remember more information about patients they have seen. Therefore, use your clinical experience as much as you can. Making up fictitious cases and hanging information, especially fine detail on this structure, is also good. If you are trying to learn a particular name of a drug for example, try and personalise it, give it a character, or add colour.

Use Memory Aids

Make it task-specific. Look at the structure of the information. For example, if it is a process, then make a flow chart, or make up a story. If it is a polysyllabic word or an anatomical label, break it into syllables and use a colour-coding system. Memory and recall work best if you exaggerate and elaborate on what is being learned make it funny or personalise it. It is also important to keep a record of what you have achieved and review and evaluate it regularly. The review does not need to be in-depth, unless you really cannot remember the information, but it makes knowledge more readily accessible.

Strategies for the Exams – Plan, Prepare, and Practice

Success in an exam at this level is more likely if you feel ready for it. If the revision plan has gone well, then you should be feeling as confident as you can in your knowledge. Most medical exams have a vast curriculum, and given the demanding job that you do, it is unrealistic to think you can know it all. There is an element of luck in these exams, but good preparation and practice can mitigate this.

Preparation involves practising exam questions, but a note of caution – just doing questions is often not enough to pass, especially for dyslexic people. Dyslexic people need to understand and reprocess the material so they can recall it more easily. They learn it more thoroughly because rote learning will not work. They may take longer and do more re-sits, but arguably, dyslexic doctors who have failed exams on several occasions may have more knowledge than doctors who pass the first time; they can be better doctors, and they can have more confidence because of that knowledge.

Nevertheless, practising questions is important for two reasons. Firstly, you familiarise yourself with the knowledge required and with the way the questions are phrased. It helps to think strategically and try to understand why the question is being asked, why it is important, and what the examiners are trying to assess.

Secondly, if you practice doing questions at speed, the same speed as you need to in the exam, e.g. 20 questions in 30 minutes, you are practising reading and recalling at pace – which is what the exam requires. Building this up into three sets of 30 minutes and then four sets of timed questions means you are building your cognitive stamina. You are preparing yourself for the mental marathon of the exam and familiarising yourself with the performance in the day.

Planning and being prepared about what you are going to do on the day can also help get you in the 'exam mindset'. It includes what to wear, what to eat, how to spend the time before and between the exam to combat nerves, and what to do if you get anxious (e.g. breathe deeply); being pragmatic and moving on are positive options. Exams can be harder for dyslexic people; it is not the format in which you can demonstrate your knowledge best. Knowing that you have the skills, abilities, and knowledge to do the job and that your patients and colleagues value what you do is something that can boost your self-belief, and this leads to success.

Conclusion

This chapter has outlined the complexity of dyslexia and its impact on adulthood. It is characterised by information processing difficulties that can become more evident when the demands of life and work increase. It can take a while to come to terms with and develop new skills. A diagnosis should provide an explanation for the difficulties but also outline the strengths and lead to better self-understanding and finding solutions. Exams and some aspects of the workplace, especially heavy administrative demands, are more of a challenge for dyslexic people, but this means you need to be more creative in your problem-solving: *How can I best do this?*

Being dyslexic is not a barrier to a successful career in medicine. In fact, being dyslexic means that you bring more to the role, you are unlikely to put your patients at risk because you double-check, and you always aim to do a good job.

References

1. Snowling, M.J. (2014). Dyslexia: A language learning impairment. *Journal of the British Academy, 2,* 43–58. doi: 10.5871/jba/002.043
2. McLoughlin, D. and Leather, C.A. (2013). *The adult dyslexic: Interventions and outcomes – An evidence-based approach* (2nd ed.). Chichester: John Wiley & Sons, Ltd.
3. Protopapa, C. and Smith-Spark, J.H. (2022). Self-reported symptoms of developmental dyslexia predict impairments in everyday cognition in adults. *Research in Developmental Disabilities, 128,* 104288.
4. Gerber, P.J., Ginsberg, R., and Reiff, H.B. (1992). Identifying alterable patterns in employment success for highly successful adults with learning

disabilities. *Journal of Learning Disabilities*, 25(8), 475–487. Available from: https://journals-sagepub-com.ezp-prod1.hul.harvard.edu/doi/abs/10.1177/002221949202500802

5. Madaus, J.W., Zhao, J., and Ruban, L. (2008). Employment satisfaction of university graduates with learning disabilities. *Remedial and Special Education*, 29(6), 323–332. Available from: https://journals-sagepub-com.ezp-prod1.hul.harvard.edu/doi/abs/10.1177/0741932507312012

6. Schnieders, C.A., Gerber, P.J., and Goldberg, R.J. (2016). Integrating findings of studies of successful adult with learning disabilities: A new comprehensive model for researchers and practitioners. *Career Planning and Adult Development Journal*, 31(4), 90–110.

7. Leather, C., Hogh, H., Seiss, E., and Everatt, J. (2011). Cognitive functioning and work success in adults with dyslexia. *Dyslexia*, 17(4), 327–338. Available from: https://onlinelibrary-wiley-com.ezp-prod1.hul.harvard.edu/doi/full/10.1002/dys.441

8. Miles, T.R. and Miles, E. (1990). *Dyslexia: A hundred years on*. Milton Keynes: Open University Press.

9. *The Dyslexia Handbook 2021*.

10. Frith, U. (1999). Paradoxes in the definition of dyslexia. *Dyslexia*, 5, 192–214.

11. Shaywitz, S.E. (2003). Overcoming dyslexia: A new and complete science-based program for reading problems at any level [cited 2023 May 7], 416. Available from: https://www.barnesandnoble.com/w/overcoming-dyslexia-sally-shaywitz-md/1133983833

12. Smythe, I. and British Dyslexia Association. (2001). *The dyslexia handbook, 2001: A compendium of articles, checklists, resources and contacts for dyslexic people, their families and teachers*.

13. Martin, A.E. and McLoughlin, D. (2012). Disclosing dyslexia: An exercise in self-advocacy. In N. Brunswick (Ed.), *Supporting dyslexic adults in higher education and the workplace*. Chichester: Wiley, 125–135.

14. Kinsella, M., Waduud, M.A., and Biddlestone, J. (2017). Dyslexic doctors, an observation on current United Kingdom practice. *MedEdPublish*, 6, 60.

15. Asghar, Z., Williams, N., Denney, M., and Siriwardena, A.N. (2019). Performance in candidates declaring versus those not declaring dyslexia in a licensing clinical examination. *Medical Education*, 53(12), 1243–1252. Available from: https://onlinelibrary.wiley.com/doi/full/10.1111/medu.13953

16. Doyle, N. and McDowall, A. (2015). Is coaching an effective adjustment for dyslexic adults? *Coaching: An International Journal of Theory, Research & Practice*, 8(2), 154–168.

17. Flinn, F. and Armstrong, C. (2011). Junior doctors' extended work hours and the effects on their performance: The Irish case. *International Journal for Quality in Health Care*, 23(2), 210–217. Available from: https://academic-oup-com.ezp-prod1.hul.harvard.edu/intqhc/article/23/2/210/1786502

chapter twenty

Out in Surgery – LGBTQ Issues

Mustafa Khanbhai

Not Quite over the Rainbow

Many lesbian, gay, bisexual, transgender, and queer (LGBTQ) doctors continue to find their workplace to be a challenging environment as they routinely encounter discrimination from colleagues, staff, and patients, which leaves them feeling uncomfortable and unwelcome (1). Although evidence suggests that the climate of acceptance has improved over the last quarter-century, LGBTQ doctors still experience or fear overt discrimination.

A 2016 survey conducted by the British Medical Association (BMA), in conjunction with the Association of LGBTQ Doctors and Dentists (GLADD) (2), found that respondents felt uncomfortable in the environment they were working in and experienced homophobic abuse, harassment, and discrimination in employment or education. Across the Atlantic, a similar survey conducted by Eliason et al. (3) reported that LGBTQ doctors experienced being denied privileges, promotions, employment, and patient referrals and face workplace harassment and social exclusion.

Closeted Operating Theatres

Sadly, the experiences of LGBTQ doctors are not uniform across specialities, with surgical specialities historically having more conservative working environments (4). A recent study (5) uncovered the challenges associated with LGBTQ equality and inclusion, with surgical trainees significantly more likely to experience workplace discrimination, harassment, and bullying and twice as likely to consider leaving their program.

These alarming facts are not isolated to surgical trainees. When surveyed (6) about medical speciality choice and perceived inclusivity toward sexual and gender minority groups, medical students reported surgery to be least inclusive. The perceived lack of inclusivity in surgery impedes the recruitment of LGBTQ trainees into surgical training and poses the risk of missing opportunities to address the unique needs and healthcare disparities present within the LGBTQ community (7). LGBTQ trainees must expend considerable energy constantly assessing their environments,

DOI: 10.1201/9781003350422-21

struggling to find a balance between self-protection and self-disclosure; this energy represents a net loss to surgical training programs and the profession (8).

Embracing a Surgical Gaydar

In the United Kingdom, there has been a positive change to address some of the challenges facing LGBTQ surgeons. In 2021, the Royal College of Surgeons of England (RCSEng) commissioned an independent review (9), led by Baroness Helena Kennedy, QC, into the diversity of the leadership of the surgical profession and of the College. The report concluded that the RCS is short on diversity and inclusion and is out of step with our society and the changing profession of surgery. In addition to the 16-point action plan from the report, the RCSE chose to develop an LGBTQ strategy encouraging a culture of upstanders rather than bystanders.

Following on from this report, on 25 March 2022, for the first time since the inception of the RCSEng in 1800, the RCSEng held a conference bringing together LGBTQ surgeons and allies in collaboration with Pride in Surgery Forum (PRiSM), which is now part of the RCSEng network of LGBTQ surgeons and allies providing visibility, role models, and an association. This move was in the right direction, demonstrating acceptance and progress in ensuring LGBT surgeons have a voice.

In September 2022, the Intercollegiate Committee for Basic Surgical Examinations (ICBSE) of the Surgical Royal Colleges of the United Kingdom and Ireland apologised for an inappropriate question in the Intercollegiate MRCS Part A exam that was rooted in homophobic prejudice. Various doctors on social media voiced their concerns, and the ICBSE agreed that it was poorly worded and caused offence.

There is still much to be accomplished within the surgical community to create a more equitable and inclusive environment for all LGBTQ surgeons. However, actively addressing issues raised and improving the diversity within surgery is not simply a bandwagon the RCSEng has joined but is important for the future of the profession, in terms of workforce, innovation, and surgical talent. Healthcare organisations are also embracing change and creating a workplace where everyone feels valued – for example, by introducing the option for employees to have their pronouns included alongside their names.

Only by challenging the stereotypes that have existed for so long can surgery grow and continue to attract the most talented individuals from medical schools. There is a growing movement and changes in policy that have facilitated our voice to be heard so that LGBTQ surgeons who have not previously felt comfortable being out at work can see it is now possible.

Prideful Resources

The resources available to LGBTQ surgeons are few and far between. Some of the organisations listed here are working hard to change the status quo:

- The Association of LGBTQ+ Doctors and Dentists (GLADD) – https://gladd.co.uk
- Pride in Surgery Forum (PRiSM) – @PRiSM_Surgery
- Association of Out Surgeons and Allies (AOSA) – @OutSurgeons
- Gay and Lesbian Medical Association (GLMA) – www.glma.org
- Pride Ortho – https://prideortho.org

Most healthcare organisations now have a webpage dedicated to LGBTQ resources, including support on their social media platforms, which demonstrates progress towards inclusivity.

Born This Way – Case Study: Mustafa Khanbhai

I am currently a speciality registrar in Oncoplastic Breast surgery with a portfolio career. I have completed a PhD and hold two fellowships as a clinical entrepreneur and in clinical artificial intelligence. I am openly gay with my friends and some of the junior doctors but stop short of being fully open at work. It has taken me a while to trust people before being open, and every time I started a rotation, there was always a fear in the back of my mind that people would see and treat me differently if they found out about my sexuality. I have been very aware of the hierarchy in surgery, where I felt more comfortable being open with nurses and other junior doctors but reluctant to disclose my sexual orientation to anyone senior. I was fearful that being honest about my sexuality would lead to negative repercussions with respect to career progression and jeopardise my opportunities by letting my personal life spill over too much. When moving to a different organisation as part of my surgical training, I was always a little concerned that I would be allocated to a supervisor who may have implicit, deeply ingrained beliefs on cisgender heteronormative societal ideas. Similarly, many LGBTQ doctors feel pressure to conceal their identities from co-workers and patients due to explicit and implicit prejudice. Many doctors have to live with the stress of being 'outed' when trying to conceal their LGBTQ identity, thereby damaging personal integrity, workplace community, and productivity (10).

Occasionally hearing homophobic banter in the surgical workplace, which sometimes had an undertone of malice, made social interactions at work very challenging. This affected my interactions at work, where I would ensure there was minimal conversation about my life outside of work, and if the conversation headed that way, I would change the subject immediately. I suspect some of my colleagues would have perceived me as being frosty as I did not talk about my private life. Perhaps this was because I still felt that much of my inhibition was coming from myself rather than from the wider team. Mainly, I do not want people to feel uncomfortable.

Overall, I have generally had a positive response about my sexuality from my immediate surgical team in most rotations. Particularly during the latter end of my career, I felt the teams I worked with let me be my true authentic self at work. I was able to achieve more and be able to function better at work and emerge successful. This is in keeping with evidence from the United States where LGBTQ respondents reported the same levels of satisfaction with their decision to become surgeons (5). This suggests that promoting an inclusive and equitable environment can be very effective in retaining LGBTQ surgeons and increasing their level of personal dignity and job satisfaction.

Personally, I have seen a change in attitudes towards homosexuality during my career and now feel that surgery and the NHS are good places for LGBTQ people to progress in. I hope this demonstrates to prospective trainees and medical students that it is indeed feasible to both be yourself and have a surgical career. I hope to continue to contribute to our surgical profession in a positive manner, and I am grateful to be given this opportunity to do so.

References

1. Burke BP, White JC. The well-being of gay, lesbian, and bisexual physicians. *West J Med*. 2001;174(1):59–62.
2. https://nwpgmd.nhs.uk/sites/default/files/Experience-of-LGB-doctors-and-medical-students%20in%20NHS-v9.pdf.
3. Eliason MJ, Dibble SL, Robertson PA. Lesbian, gay, bisexual, and transgender (LGBT) physicians' experiences in the workplace. *J Homosex*. 2011;58(10): 1355–71. doi: 10.1080/00918369.2011.614902. PMID: 22029561.
4. Ramos MM, Téllez CM, Palley TB, Umland BE, Skipper BJ. Attitudes of physicians practicing in New Mexico toward gay men and lesbians in the profession. *Acad Med*. 1998;73(4):436–8.
5. Heiderscheit EA, Schlick CJR, Ellis RJ, et al. Experiences of LGBTQ+ Residents in US general surgery training programs. *JAMA Surg*. 2021;157(14):e215246.
6. Sitkin NA, Pachankis JE. Specialty choice among sexual and gender minorities in medicine: The role of specialty prestige, perceived inclusion, and medical school climate. *LGBT Health*. 2016;3(6):451–60.
7. Quinn GP, Sanchez JA, Sutton SK, et al. Cancer and lesbian, gay, bisexual, transgender/transsexual, and queer/questioning (LGBTQ) populations: Cancer and sexual minorities. *CA Cancer J Clin*. 2015;65(5):384–400.

8. Risdon C, Cook D, Willms D. Gay and lesbian physicians in training: A qualitative study. *CMAJ*. 2000;162(3):331–4.

9. www.rcseng.ac.uk/about-the-rcs/about-our-mission/diversity-review-2021/.

10. Lee KP, Kelz RR, Dubé B, Morris JB. Attitude, and perceptions of the other underrepresented minority in surgery. *J Surg Educ*. 2014;71(6):e47–e52.

Chapter twenty one

Getting into Core Surgical Training as an Ethnic Minority

Tolu Ekong, Temitope Ajala-Agbo, and Eniola Salau

Representation matters! You probably read a story of how someone was inspired to accomplish something great because they saw someone like them do it first. The challenge with minority groups is that such role models are hard to find. If you are a future surgical trainee from a minority group, this is a reality you will in all probability face.

On the other side of the coin, there are patients. Being admitted to a hospital is a scary prospect. Having surgery is even scarier. Having a surgeon who looks like you and understands your cultural norms can go a long way in putting the patient at ease during a stressful time. So if you are an ethnic minority and interested in surgery, you are very much needed.

The population of the United Kingdom is around 68 million of which about 87% are white British. The approximate breakdown of the minority ethnic groups is shown in Table 21.1.

You may not be aware of the following statistic, but as an ethnic minority, compared with your Caucasian colleagues, you are more than twice as likely to fail your professional exams[1, 2] and to be unsuccessful in gaining a core or speciality training position in your desired speciality,[3] especially if your desired speciality is a surgical one. And this is despite having been trained in a UK medical school and accounting for other contributory factors. For the black trainee, even when you do get into core or speciality training, the attrition rate is about 50%; only half of the total number of black trainees make it to consultant grade, as shown in Table 21.2. The conversion rate from trainee to consultant as a black female surgical trainee is even worse.[4] There are several theories as to why this may be the case, although no one truly understands the dynamics and the magnitude of the effect each factor has.

The observed difference in performance between ethnic minority groups and their white counterparts has been termed 'differential attainment'. Differential attainment was first reported in 1995[5] where several factors, including biased examiners and learner deficits, were blamed for this phenomenon at first. However, studies which have taken into account these

DOI: 10.1201/9781003350422-22

Table 21.1 UK Population Data (https://populationdata.
org.uk/uk-population/)

	Percentage
White British	87
Asian/Asian British	7
Black/Black British	3
Mixed/multiple ethnic groups	2
Other ethnic groups	1

Table 21.2 Percentage of NHS Medical Staff by Ethnicity and Broad Grade (NHS workforce statistics, www.ethnicity-facts-figures.service.gov.uk/workforce-and-business/workforce-diversity/nhs-workforce/latest – published Feb. 2020, updated Aug 2020)

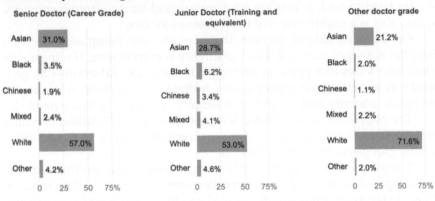

factors and others have shown that there is a lot more to the significant difference observed in the performance of ethnic minority groups in medicine.

There is evidence that interactions with peers and superiors are significant in affecting career outcomes.[6] The social aspect of learning and, therefore, the learning experience of ethnic minority groups are believed to play a major role in the differential attainment observed.[7] A review found that minority medical students 'experienced less supportive social and less positive learning environments and were subject to discrimination and racial harassment.'[8] Medical students and trainees learn best from teachers who support, believe in, and invested in them. This in itself is a predictor of career success.[9, 10]

In our opinion, a combination of factors contributes to these statistical findings, and there is more research to be done on the matter. The recent spotlight on equality and diversity has forced several organisations, including the General Medical Council (GMC) and Royal College of Surgeons (RCS), among many others, to pay attention to differential attainment. A lot of work is already being done by these organisations to create awareness and a culture change towards equality and diversity. Nevertheless, much work and time are required to change the given statistic for *you* who are planning to successfully apply for Core Surgical Training.

So what can *you* do to increase your chances of realising your dreams of becoming a surgeon? Well, you can lay hold of the experiences, both good and bad, of those who have gone before you and learn from them. An increasing number of ethnic minorities are gaining places in surgical specialities and having successful surgical careers. So what did they do and continue to do to make this possible? I have identified some personality traits and actions common in those that have been successful in this path. Let us review them here.

Have a Solid Plan

Do not become indecisive because you are suffering with imposter syndrome and feel like no one looks like you in the surgical world. Of course, there are not many people that look like you in surgery. Have you read and digested the given stats yet? This is why you must push through and become an example to the next cohort.

It is never too early to start planning. The plotting and planning begin from the first moment you had thought of being a surgeon. You need to learn to play the game and 'speak surgery'. There are certain hoops you have to jump through whether you like it or not. So roll your sleeves up and get jumping!

Make sure you set yourself up to be known in the surgical community. Network with other students that have chosen surgery as their career path (I know they can be annoying at times, but trust me, you need them). That is how you get the latest tips and find opportunities to be involved in regional and national projects. Think about taking on leadership positions in your medical school's surgical society or similar university-based organisations.

Be part of national organisations that promote and support ethnic minorities in medicine and surgery, such as the British Association of Physicians of Indian Origin (BAPIO), UK Black Surgeons Network (UKBSN), British Association of Black Surgeons (BABS), and Melanin Medics. These organisations are also good places for networking and finding mentors.

Surgical Mentorship and Sponsorship

Find an inspiring role model you admire and ask them to mentor you. Surgical registrars often make the best mentors for medical students and junior doctors. They have been where you are and are not too far removed to give sound advice. They are often more approachable. If you find someone whom you like to guide you along the way, reach out to them, and they will be flattered and even keen to pass on their insights – trust me! If you cannot find anyone in your hospital, try social media. Look on Instagram, Twitter, LinkedIn, etc. This is the one time it is okay to stalk!

The role of mentorship in surgery cannot be underestimated. There are people who have successfully walked the path you are on or about to take. They can guide you. Your role model does not have to look like you; they just have to care enough about your progress and be invested in your success. Sometimes a mentor is for a season; other times, they are for life. It may take a while to find a mentor you gel well with, but when you do, hold on to them tight. Ensure you have a mentor for every stage of your career.

Believe in Yourself

Get a life or career coach if necessary! You are good enough. You have what it takes. Now you just have to believe it. I have noticed a pattern of lack of self-belief with medical students/doctors of ethnic minority backgrounds. That can adversely impact your performance. So although the audit, research publications, and presentations are important, it is a good idea to invest in building your sense of self. Know who you are, your strengths, and your weaknesses, and understand your likes and dislikes. Take personality tests to better understand yourself. Get a coach if necessary to work through some of your self-doubts. Confidence is key, and your Caucasian colleagues already have one up on you here; just being 'the only' in the room, which I am sure you often are, puts you on the back foot. So be proactive with this one.

Be True to Yourself

Bring all of you. Diversity really is needed in the surgical speciality. It is not just a slogan or a matter of fulfilling the ethnic minority quota. Our patients are diverse and need a diverse group of surgeons. It is not just about colour. A lot of ethnic minorities try to fit into the stereotypical surgical mould. I certainly did so. But after years of trying to fit in, I realised that my uniqueness made me special and added value to my patients, my colleagues, and even my superiors. By being yourself, you bring a different way of thinking into the workplace for the good of all; marginalised groups are more likely to engage with healthcare services if they feel that they can identify with their physician.[11] Katherine Phillips, in her research, found that diversity breeds empathy and better cognitive reasoning. Interestingly, she found that just the presence of an ethnic minority in a team, without them having to speak, causes a diversity of thinking for the better.[12]

Be Creative

Do not put yourself in a box. As medics in general, we can lack creativity, or rather the study and demands of medicine beat the creativity out of us! Feed your creativity; invest in your hobbies outside of medicine. Hang out with non-medics. Think outside of the surgical box and the well-trodden path taken by other medical students/junior doctors. Take out time to pursue other interests, but be sure to creatively link them to your chosen surgical speciality, and even if you cannot, exploring other interests for a season really does make you a well-rounded individual. No one wants a boring surgeon as a colleague!

Speak Up and Take Opportunities

As ethnic minorities, we can sometimes be found wanting in this area. Do not shrink back! A senior colleague is talking about a project they are involved with over team coffee. Be bold and speak up. Ask to join in. That project could become your first presentation or publication. What is the worst that could happen? They say no, and you move on. Be keen and be diligent in everything you do at work; stand out as the responsible and reliable member of any team you find yourself in. Pay additional attention to detail. Be kind, and get to know everyone in your sphere of influence, from the clerk, cleaner, porter, and nurses on your ward to your clinical supervisors, clinical directors, and even the chief executive of your trust. It goes a long way!

Community and Family Support

Build a community around you. These people do not have to be surgeons or medics; they just have to have your back! Surgical training is a marathon, and you definitely need cheerleaders along the way to emotionally support you when the going gets tough. Do not cast aside valuable relationships in the pursuit of a surgical career. Rather, invest in strategic relationships; you will be better for it. If you are a person of faith, plunge deeper into your faith; it can only serve you well.

Keep the End Goal in Mind!

Keep the end in focus. There is life beyond training. Do not get distracted by side shows! Ruthlessly eliminate time wasters in your life. As you go further in your training, you will encounter several demotivating situations. You may experience personal or family illness, bullying, sexism, poor training, and so on. Build your resilience and prepare for the possibility of such situations so that they do not knock you off course. You have come too far and sacrificed too much to let some bully take your dream away.

For those who choose to start a family during training, it is particularly difficult as your parental instincts will pull you homewards while your career takes you away from your family. Your training may be extended if you become a parent, so prepare to see your colleagues move ahead of you for a season, but it will be okay because you have kept the end goal in mind!

And finally . . .

Lift as You Climb

Remember to send the *ladder* down for others. By virtue of your success, you are a change agent for others. Choose to be an active change agent. The platform you have is exactly what is needed to change the statistics given and make it easier for the next generation.

References

1. General Medical Council. The state of medical education and practice in the UK. General Medical Council, 2015. Google Scholar.
2. Woolf K, Potts HWW, McManus IC. Ethnicity and academic performance in UK trained doctors and medical students: Systematic review and meta-analysis. BMJ 2011;342:d901. doi:10.1136/bmj.d901
3. Lacobucci G. Specialty training: Ethnic minority doctors' reduced chance of being appointed is "unacceptable." BMJ 2020;368:m479.
4. Woodhams C, Parnerkar I, Tomaskovic-Devey D. Relational inequalities in UK surgery: Gender, race and closure. Acad Manag Proc 2022;(1). doi:10.5465/AMBPP.2022.239
5. Dillner L. Manchester tackles failure rate of Asian students. BMJ 1995;310:209. doi:10.1136/bmj.310.6974.209
6. Schneider M, Preckel F. Variables associated with achievement in higher education: A systematic review of meta-analyses. Psychol Bull 2017;143:565–600. doi:10.1037/bul0000098
7. Woolf K, Potts HWW, Patel S, McManus IC. The hidden medical school: A longitudinal study of how social networks form, and how they relate to academic performance. MedTeach 2012;34:577–586. doi:10.3109/0142159X.2012.669082
8. Orom H, Semalulu T, Underwood W 3rd. The social and learning environments experienced by underrepresented minority medical students: A narrative review. Acad Med 2013;88:1765–1777. doi:10.1097/ACM.0b013e3182a7a3af
9. Woolf K, Rich A, Viney R, Needleman S, Griffin A. Perceived causes of differential attainment in UK postgraduate medical training: A national qualitative study. BMJ Open 2016;6:e013429. doi:10.1136/bmjopen-2016-013429

10. Ng TWH, Eby LT, Sorensen KL, Feldman DC. Predictors of objective and subjective career success: A meta-analysis. Person Psychol 2005;58:367–408. doi:10.1111/j.1744-6570.2005.00515.x

11. Butler PD, Aarons CB, Ahn J, Wein AJ, Ruckenstein MJ, Lett LA, DeMatteo RP, Serletti, JM. Leading from the front. Ann Surg 2019;269(6):1012–1015. doi:10.1097/SLA.0000000000003197

12. Phillips K, Northcraft G, Neale M. Stanford university surface-level diversity R and decision-making in groups: When does deep-level similarity help? Group Processes Intergroup Relat 2006;9(4):467–482.

Index

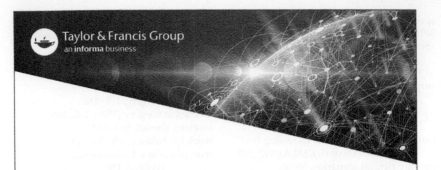